Drug Treatment
in the Elderly

Drug Treatment in the Elderly

Elspeth T. Macdonald
Lately Associate Specialist,
Department of Health Care of the Elderly,
Sherwood Hospital, Nottingham

and

J. B. Macdonald
Consultant Physician,
North Ayrshire District General Hospital,
Kilmarnock, and Ayrshire Central Hospital,
Irvine, Scotland

A Wiley Medical Publication

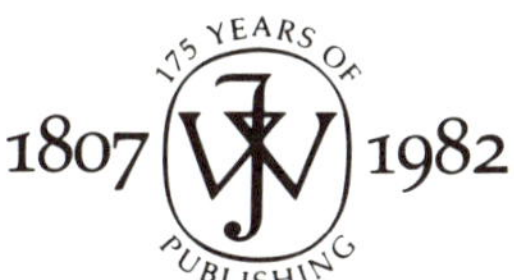

JOHN WILEY & SONS
Chichester · New York · Brisbane · Toronto · Singapore

Library of Congress Cataloging in Publication Data:
Macdonald, Elspeth T.
    Drug treatment in the elderly.
    (Wiley series on disease management in the elderly;
v. 1) (A Wiley medical publication)
    Includes index.
    1. Geriatric pharmacology. I. Macdonald, J. B.
II. Title.   III. Series.   IV. Series: Wiley medical
publication.   [DNLM: 1. Drug therapy—In old age.
W1 WI53M v. 1 / WT 100 M135d]
RC953.7.M253   615.5′8′0880565   82–1913

ISBN 0 471 10216 4   AACR2

British Library Cataloging in Publication Data:
Drug treatment in the elderly.—(Disease management
    in the elderly; v. 1).—(A Wiley medical publication)
    1. Geriatric pharmacology
    I. Macdonald, Elspeth T.   II. Macdonald, J. B.
    III. Series
    615.5′8   RC953.7

ISBN 0 471 10216 4

Photoset by Paston Press, Norwich
Printed by Pitman Press Ltd., Bath, Avon

Contents

Acknowledgements

We wish to record our indebtedness to Dr A. Fairley, who kindled our interest in drug problems in the elderly. We also thank Mrs M. Gammie, Mrs A. Murdoch and Miss K. Leitch for invaluable secretarial help. We are also most grateful for the tolerance and support of Dr J. Jarvis (John Wiley & Sons).

Series preface

In 1881 the clinical lectures of the great French physician Jean–Marie Charcot on senile and chronic diseases were translated and published in English. In these lectures he emphasized the importance of studying the pathology of the diseases of old age claiming that only by such careful study would these diseases be clearly understood. In other words he was saying, 'What happens?', 'Why does it happen?', and 'How can we put it right?'

Geriatric Medicine is a comparatively new specialty. There were only four consultant physicians in Geriatric Medicine when the NHS started in 1948. In 1981 the number has expanded to exceed 500 and if the recommendations of the Short report are implemented, the number may well exceed 800. Such an expansion could not have occurred if those who practice in the specialty did not achieve satisfaction from their work. As Charcot pointed out, this is a 'very interesting part of medicine'. Doctors and others who are working in the field of the elderly have become fascinated by the 'What?' and 'Why?' and 'How?'.

As a result a discipline with its own body of knowledge has developed. That this body of knowledge exists has even been recognized by the Education Committee of the General Medical Council in 1980 when, in issuing new recommendations concerning the undergraduate medical curriculum, it emphasized that the 'attention of the student should be constantly directed to . . . the growing importance of the problems posed by disability and disease in an increasingly elderly population', and 'should receive instruction in the special problems and diagnosis and treatment of illness in the elderly . . .'

Sir William Osler once wrote that to study medicine without books is like sailing the sea without a chart. The same applies to Geriatric Medicine. Many excellent books have already been written on the subject. The specialty though, is still developing and our knowledge of the 'What, why and how?' is expanding. As Charcot said, 'its difficulties can only be surmounted by long experience and a profound knowledge of its peculiar characters'.

In this series of books concerning disease management in the elderly, the Authors and Editors have tried to draw on their experience and knowledge to attempt to answer some of the questions posed by What? Why? and How? in relation to the topics which they have chosen. It is hoped that the series will help students of Geriatric Medicine, whether they be undergraduates or postgraduate doctors or students or practitioners in the professions complementary to medicine such as nursing and remedial therapy, to a greater understanding of illness in the elderly. If this hope is achieved then some of the difficulties posed by 'senile pathology' may be surmounted so that those elderly may be enabled to lead fuller and more active lives.

M. R. P. HALL
Professor of Geriatric Medicine,
University of Southampton

Introduction

The aged are a very special group with relation to drugs. Their ability to handle drugs is altered. Multiple pathology is the rule rather than the exception. In paediatric practice great care is taken to emphasize dosage alterations. It is a great pity that such care is not taken with the elderly, thereby avoiding much needless morbidity and even mortality.

The problem of drug use in the elderly is large and growing steadily. At present in the United Kingdom there are some 7.5 million people over the age of 65 years. Of this group 2.7 million are over the age of 75 years and 450,000 are over the age of 85 years. It has also been estimated that 20% of the population over 80 years is severely demented (Editorial, 1981). The annual NHS expenditure on drugs is around £1000m (of which at least £40m is spent on drugs which are never taken). Of this enormous drug budget some 30% is taken up by patients over 65 years (Crooks *et al.*, 1975). This huge consumption of drugs produces some horrendous statistics: 75% of the population over the age of 75 years is on regular medication. Two-thirds of these regular drug-users take one to three drugs daily, while one-third take four to six drugs regularly (Skegg *et al.*, 1977; Williamson, 1978). Skegg and his co-workers (1977) estimated that 37% of all women over the age of 75 years receive regular therapy with psychotropic drugs. By far the most unpalatable statistic is that 10% of all admissions to geriatric units are directly due to drug-induced disease (Williamson, 1978). Hurwitz and Wade (1969) and Seidl *et al.* (1966) also found that the incidence of adverse drug reactions rises sharply with age, from less than 3% in the age range 20–29 to 21% in those over 70 years. Surveys of hospital admissions naturally do not include any estimates of those large numbers of people in the community who are experiencing unnecessary suffering as a result of their medication. Here estimates are more difficult since they are altered by the misuse of drugs (e.g. pill-swapping, taking old medication, taking self-purchased proprietary preparations, etc.) (Macdonald *et al.*, 1977).

The reasons behind this vast toll of iatrogenic misery are many are varied. Drug companies often fail to appreciate that preparations for general use may be totally unsuited to the elderly subject. The medical profession often fails to understand that the altered physiology of the aged, coupled with altered pharmacokinetics and pharmacodynamics, provide a potent trap for the unwary.

Many cynical geriatricians state that their greatest therapeutic successes are achieved by stopping the drugs with which their colleagues were poisoning their patients. It is the clear responsibility of those prescribing for the elderly, indeed prescribing for anyone, to have a clear understanding of the pharmacological actions of every drug they prescribe. Those prescribing for the elderly need a sound grasp of how drug effects are altered by the changes in body function with age and disease. Symptoms in the elderly are often vague and misleading. Disaster is often the result when treatment is started in the absence of a sound diagnosis. It is also essential to remember that drugs are not a cure for social or economic conditions.

In this volume it is proposed to consider the particular problems of the elderly patient in three main groupings. Section One deals with the alterations in physiology associated with ageing and the way in which drug handling is altered by these changes. Section Two will consider the use of drugs in various clinical situations. Here drugs are grouped by body system. This section does not claim to be comprehensive. Conditions have been included either because they are common or because therapy carries particular hazards in the elderly patient. Section Three deals with events after the prescription—patient compliance, prescribing habits, packaging etc.—and how these can contribute to drug problems in the elderly.

Where pharmocological research data are immediately relevant, these have been included. However, the main aim of the book is to clarify some of the everyday difficulties in prescribing for older people.

REFERENCES

Crooks, J. *et al*. (1975) Drugs and the elderly: the nature of the problem. *Health Bulletin*, **33**, 222–7.

Editorial (1981) Organic mental impairment in the elderly. *Lancet*, **2**, 561.

Hurwitz, N. and Wade, O. (1969) Intensive hospital monitoring of adverse hospital reactions to drugs. *Brit. Med. J.*, **1**, 531–9.

Macdonald, E. T. *et al*. (1977) Methods of improving compliance after hospital discharge. *Brit. Med. J.*, **2**, 618–21.

Seidl, L. G. *et al*. (1966) Studies on the epidemiology of adverse drug reactions. *Bull. Johns Hopkins Hosp.*, **119**, 299–315.

Skegg, D. C. G., Doll, R., and Perry, J. (1977) Use of medicines in general practice. *Brit. Med. J.*, **1**, 1561–3.

Williamson, J. (1978) Prescribing problems in the elderly. *Practitioner*, **220**, 749–55.

Section One

Chapter 1

The physiology of ageing

We are all familiar with the external manifestations of old age—the stooped posture, wrinkled skin, grey hair and spectacles. More important are the changes caused by decline in function of the vital organs. These changes will be considered systematically and the main physiological changes are summarized in Table 1.1. There are, however, a few general points which need to be detailed first.

With advancing age there are general histological changes which take place throughout the body tissue. Cells are lost and the remainder tend to enlarge, resulting in increasing irregularity of the tissue architecture. It has been estimated that the total number of body cells decreases by 30% between 25 years and 70 years (Goldman, 1971). The decrease in the total mass of active cells is accompanied by an identical decrease in the basal oxygen consumption (Shock *et al.*, 1953). A similar decrease occurs in total body protein and intracellular water (Lesser *et al.*, 1963 and Moore *et al.*, 1963), but extracellular water and plasma volume remain constant (Edelman and Leibman, 1959). A significant sex difference in mean body water content appears at puberty and persists throughout life. It has been shown to be due primarily to the difference in body fat content (Forbes and Reina, 1970). The alterations in the main body components are shown in Figure 1.1.

There is also a decline in both the absolute and relative body potassium. This too is best explained by an increase in relative fat content and a decrease in lean body mass (Forbes and Reina, 1970). The rate of decline of lean body mass accelerates with the years. By 65–70 years men have 12 kg less than at 25 years, while for women the figure is only 5 kg.

Regional blood perfusion diminishes, partly due to decreased tissue demand and partly due to alterations in the vascular supply network (Landowne and Stanley, 1960).

In some instances the overall tissue unit remains intact but become less efficient. Perhaps the best example of this is the increasing delay in the neuronal conduction time in the peripheral nervous system.

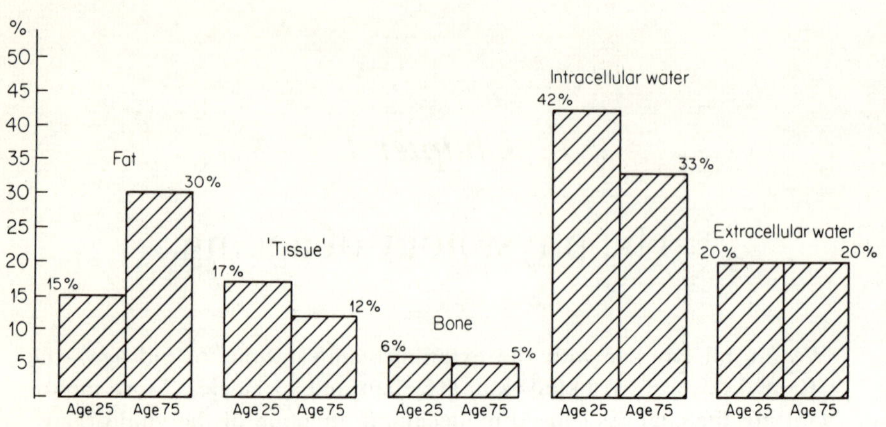

Fig. 1.1   Alteration in the main body components with age

CARDIOVASCULAR SYSTEM

In 1955 Brandfonbrener *et al.* produced a major study of the alterations in cardiovascular dynamics associated with ageing. Several anatomical changes gradually occur in the heart above the age of 30 years— increased pigmentation, endocardial thickening, and increased collagen and elastic fibres. These changes are usually not sufficient to cause haemodynamic upset, even in old age. The cardiac output decreases by 1% per annum and stroke volume declines by 0.7% per annum, both indices showing a cumulative decrease of 30–40% between the ages of 25 and 65 years (Brandfonbrener *et al.*, 1955). Circulation transit time increases. Heart rate is usually steady or decreases slightly as the years advance. Contraction time increases, especially during the isometric phase, resulting in increased oxygen and energy requirements (Landowne *et al.*, 1955). The net result is that the heart becomes a less efficient pump, giving a lower power output for a higher energy input. The heart becomes less able to deal with stress: maximal cardiac output declines and the recovery time after exercise lengthens (Montoye *et al.*, 1968). With exercise blood pressure rises and stroke volume attempts to increase in an effort to compensate for the decreased maximal rise in heart rate which occurs in old age (Gramath *et al.*, 1964). The resting arterial–venous oxygen difference also increases.

There are also considerable changes in the vascular tree. Peripheral vascular resistance, both systematic and pulmonary, increases with age as the vascular tree becomes more rigid. This rigidity produces a greater

Table 1.1   The main anatomical and physiological changes associated with ageing

---

Cardiovascular system
    Increased cardiac pigmentation
    Decreased cardiac output
    Decreased stroke volume
    Increased circulation transit time
    Decreased maximal cardiac output
    Increased peripheral vascular resistance

Central nervous system
    Decreased number of neurones
    Increased lipofuscin deposits
    Decreased catecholamine synthesis
    Increased mono-amine oxidase activity
    Decreased cerebral oxygen consumption
    Decreased cerebral blood flow

Respiratory system
    Decreased chest wall compliance
    Increased residual volume
    Decreased vital capacity
    Decreased FEV_1 and PEFR
    Decreased arterial pO_2
    Decreased response to hypoxia and hypercapnia
    Decreased cellular immunity

Gastrointestinal system
    Decreased hepatic and splanchnic blood flow
    Decreased hepatic oxidation
    Decreased cytochrome P450
    Decreased enzyme induction
    Decreased serum albumin
    Decreased gastric pH

Renal system
    Decreased renal blood flow
    Decreased glomerular filtration rate
    Decreased tubular cell function

Endocrine system
    Decreased peripheral utilization of glucose
    Decreased aldosterone secretion
    Decreased cortisol production
    Decreased TSH response to TRH administration (in men)
    Decreased secretion of adrenal androgens with age
    Tri-iodothyronine declines with age

---

rise in systolic than in diastolic blood pressure (Harris, 1970; Master and Lasser, 1961). Pulse wave velocity diminishes and the distribution of blood to various organs alters. Cerebral blood flow is maintained at the expense of hepatic and renal blood flow, which decrease by approximately 18% between the ages of 30 and 80 years (Ritschel, 1976; Flood *et al.*, 1967).

RENAL SYSTEM

The alterations in renal physiology are among the most important factors producing drug toxicity in the elderly. Most drugs and drug metabolities are excreted via the kidneys and impaired renal function can have disastrous effects on drug excretion. The most complete study of the effect of age on renal function was conducted by Davies and Shock (1950). Their findings have been corroborated by other smaller studies (Cockcroft and Gault, 1976; Val Pilsum and Seljeskog, 1958). The renal mass shows an age-dependent decrease of 30% (Roessle and Roulet, 1932), due to the loss of entire nephron units. The ability to compensate by tissue hypertrophy declines with age. (After nephrectomy the maximum contralateral hypertrophy falls from 50% to 30% (Addis, 1948).) A marked decrease in renal perfusion occurs with age (a 56% drop between the ages of 20 and 90 years). Glomerular filtration rate (GFR) declines from 123 to 65 ml/min/1.73 m^2 between the ages of 20 and 90 years—drug excretion shows an almost parallel decline. The reductions in the blood flow and GFR produce an increase in the filtration fraction.

Tubule cell function shows an overall decrease of about 40%. For example, glucose reabsorption declines by 48% and diodotrast secretion by 44%. These two parameters show a close relationship to the decrease in GFR. However, the other main test of tubule cell function—the excretion of para-amino-hippuric acid—does not show this close relation to GFR. Miller *et al.* (1951) concluded from these estimations that the ratio of blood flows to the excretory and supportive portions of the kidney remains constant with age, although overall perfusion declines.

Daily creatinine production is directly related to the total body store of creatine phosphate in the muscles. This store declines with age. Creatinine excretion is dependent on glomerular filtration and shows an almost linear decline with increasing age. It declines some 50% (on average from 24 to 12 mg/kg/24 h) between the third and ninth decades. Serum creatinine thus reflects the balance between two factors (production and excretion) which both decline with age. So serum creatinine need not be a good index of excretion ability; a man of 70 years and a man of 25 years may have the same serum creatinine but the 70-year-old may have only half the renal function. This factor is clearly very important in the renal excretion of drugs.

Urinary volume variations have no effect on creatinine clearance. Protein ingestion and exercise can both increase creatinine clearance in the young but both these effects diminish and finally disappear with advancing age (Val Pilsum and Seljeskog, 1958). A sex difference in serum creatinine appears around the age of 20 years and remains relatively constant throughout life. There is some evidence to suggest that patients with severe renal damage have an element of negative feedback: as the serum creatinine rises, creatinine production decreases (Goldring and Chasis, 1944; Moller *et al.*, 1928). It is not known whether age affects this feedback.

Urine specific gravity (SG) decreases with age (Flood *et al.*, 1967), from averages of 1.032 at age 25 to 1.024 at age 80. The ability to concentrate urine depends on the integrity of the tubular cell and on being able to maintain an osmotic gradient in the renal medulla. The maximum urine osmolality declines from 1040 at 20 years to 750 at 80 years. The ability of the kidney to respond to antidiuretic hormone (pitressin) also declines with age (Miller *et al.*, 1953).

Adler *et al.* (1968) found that the elderly can maintain a normal acid–base balance, but within a narrower range of adaptability. The excretion of an acid load is slower in the elderly and the depression of the serum bicarbonate is prolonged. The production of ammonia is somewhat diminished. Similar changes occur in the excretion of base loads.

GASTROINTESTINAL SYSTEM

Ageing produces several alterations in gastrointestinal and biliary function. The precise role these changes play in the handling of drugs is slowly being elucidated. The main changes in the gastrointestinal tract are detailed in Figure 1.2.

The main studies, carried out in the early 1960s by Bender (Bender, 1964, 1968), showed considerable alterations in the absorption patterns of substances absorbed by active metabolic processes (Table 1.2). However, most drugs are absorbed by passive diffusion and so far little or no evidence has been found of any age-related decline in their absorption.

HEPATIC AND BILIARY SYSTEM

As age increases the mean weight of the liver declines from approximately 1930 g in the fourth decade to 1000 g in the tenth decade (Calloway *et al.*, 1965). Hepatic histology alters with age, giving an increasing

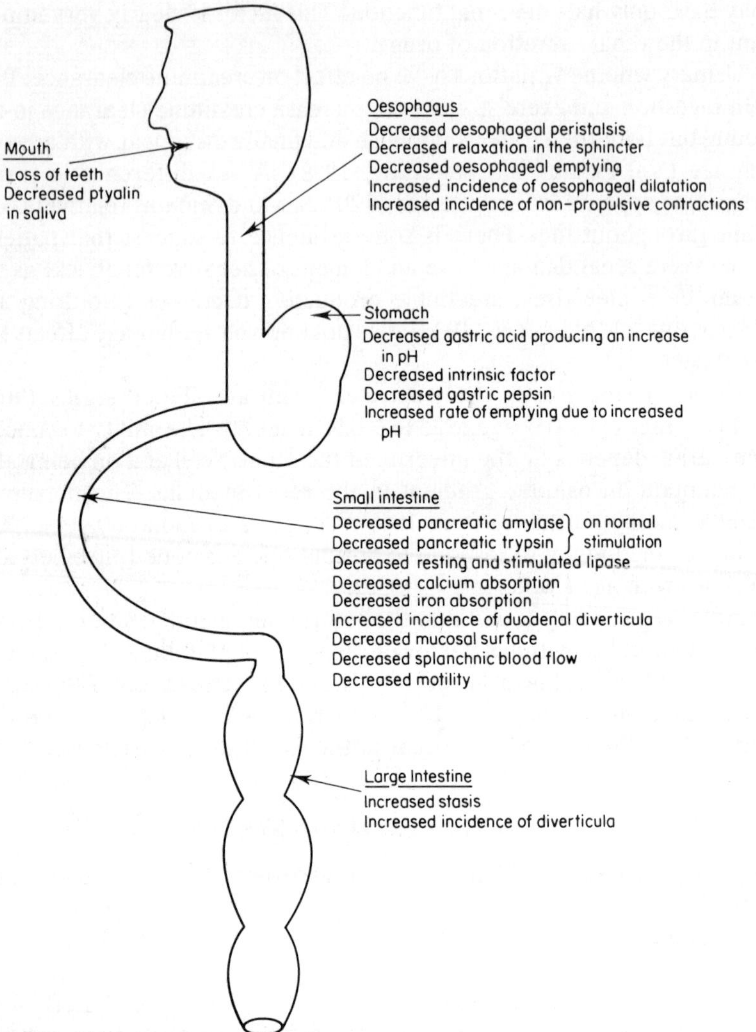

Fig. 1.2   The main changes in gastrointestinal function with age

number of giant parenchymal cells. The cell infrastructure becomes more atypical, with increasing numbers of aberrant nuclei, multiple nucleoli, nuclear inclusions and binucleate cells (Carr *et al.*, 1960).

In contrast to the histological effects of ageing the alterations in function are less well documented and the evidence at times is contradictory.

Table 1.2 Substances showing altered active absorption with age

Compound	Alteration	Points
Galactose	Delayed	
Methylcellulose	Reduced	
D-Xylose	Equivocal—normal/ reduced	
Calcium	Reduced	Thought due to decreased gastric acid
Iron	Reduced	Thought due to decreased gastric acid
Thiamine	Reduced	Animal study
Dextrose	Reduced	Animal study

Hepatic blood flow shows a significant decrease with age (0.3–1.5% per annum) (Geokas and Haverback, 1969). Where drugs are rapidly metabolized in the liver this drop in blood flow can cause a marked elevation in the serum concentration of the drug (Castleden *et al.*, 1975). Hepatic enzyme function is significantly affected by age. Hepatic microsomal oxidation which is under polygenic control (Whittaker and Evans, 1970) shows a marked reduction with age. However, acetylation, which is a non-microsomal activity under polymorphic control (Evans *et al.*, 1960), does not seem to be affected by age (Farah *et al.*, 1977). One of the most important enzymes in drug metabolism is cytochrome P450. This declines substantially with age and may contribute significantly to the higher incidence of drug reactions in the elderly. The phenomenon of enzyme induction by drugs also declines with age (Salem *et al.*, 1978).

No age-related changes in serum transaminase or bilirubin levels have been established (Kampmann *et al.*, 1975; Leask *et al.*, 1973). Leask *et al.* (1973) found an increase in the alkaline phosphatase. However, this finding has been questioned since the exclusion of people with bone disease was uncertain. An increase in bromsulphthalein (BSP) retention occurs (Freston and Englert, 1967). Thompson and Williams (1965) refined this finding and showed that age produces a liver with a reduced storage capacity but a relatively normal secretory capacity.

ENDOCRINE SYSTEM

The response to oral glucose declines by about 0.33 mmol/l per decade (Gregerman, 1967). Thus the 2 h level in a glucose tolerance test will be 1.7 mmol/l higher in a 75-year-old than in a 25-year-old. This change is

8

thought to be due to a failure in peripheral utilization of glucose. Insulin tolerance tests for growth hormone estimation can give prolonged hypoglycaemia in the elderly.

Thyroid function also shows age-related changes. Radioactive iodine accumulation in the elderly thyroid declines (Gregerman and Solomon, 1967). This appears to be due to altered renal excretion rather than any true thyroid change. The turnover rate of thyroxine decreases 50% between the ages of 20 and 80 years—from a mean of 88 μg/day at age 20 to 42 μg/day at age 80. However, the aged thyroid can respond normally to stress (Gregerman and Solomon, 1967). The response to TSH remains normal and the PBI remains unchanged. Decreased peripheral need is the most likely explanation for the changes caused by age.

The adrenals and gonads exhibit marked functional decline with age. Aldosterone excretion is reduced (Flood *et al.*, 1967). Cortisol production shows a 25% decline from a mean of 23.6 mg/day at 25 to 17.7 mg/day at 75. This is thought to be linked to the decline in muscle mass associated with ageing. There is also a decline in 17-OH corticosteroid excretion with a relatively greater decline in conjugated than unconjugated 17-OH corticosteroids.

Testosterone levels decrease with age. The relatively greater decrease in gonadal hormones compared to cortisol has been interpreted as an anabolic–catabolic imbalance giving catabolism the advantage. It has been postulated that osteoporosis may be due to the loss of the anabolic effects of the gonadal hormones. The fact that women seem to be relatively protected from atherosclerosis up to the menopause has been put forward to show the importance of the oestrogen–angrogen balance.

NERVOUS SYSTEM

Both central and peripheral nervous systems show significant alterations with age. The number of neurones declines and the weight of the brain diminishes. These changes gather momentum after the sixth decade. Cottrell (1940) found three major age-related changes in the peripheral nerves. The number of fibres decreases. The endoperineurium increases and there is progressive connective tissue infiltration of the actual nerve bundle. There are also changes in the associated vasculature: endothelial proliferation, medial fibrosis and hyalinization. Nerve conduction speed decreases.

In the central nervous system the gyri become thin and the sulci widen. This is particularly marked in the frontal and parietal regions. There is an increase in the number of fibrillary astrocytes. The nerve cell bodies show several changes: an increased lipofuscin deposition, granulo-vacuolar degeneration, neurofibrillary tangles and senile plaques. These changes tend to be most marked in the hippocampus and the limbic system (Corsellis, 1976). Davison (1978) detailed several biochemical changes found in the brain as ageing progresses: a progressive decrease in catecholamine synthesis, an increase in mono-amine oxidase activity especially in the basal ganglia and an increase in the aluminium found in the neurones.

Fazekas *et al.* (1955) studied the changes in cerebral metabolism and haemodynamics. They found a marked decline in cerebral oxygen consumption and cerebral blood flow. The special senses decline too. Visual acuity declines and dark adaptation takes longer. Acuity of hearing also decreases.

RESPIRATORY SYSTEM

In most instances the functional reserve of the lung is sufficient to compensate for the decline associated with ageing. The functional decline is less marked in women than in men. The main changes are attributable to the changes in chest wall compliance and lung compliance, although there is some decline in muscle strength (Cook *et al.*, 1964). The postural changes of kyphosis and osteroporosis combine with costal cartilage calcification and decreased rib movement to produce a decrease in chest wall compliance (Cohn and Donoso, 1963). This reduction also impairs the ability to cough. Originally it was thought that elastin within the lung increased (Pierce, 1963), making the lungs more rigid. However, it has recently been shown that elastin in the pleura increases but lung elastin remains constant (John and Thomas, 1972). Elastic recoil actually decreases with age. Wright (1961) has postulated that this is due to attenuation and decrease in the number of the elastic fibres in the alveolar ducts and mouths.

Lung volumes reflect the increasing rigidity of the rib cage and pleura. Total lung capacity and functional residual volume remain roughly constant, but residual volume increases by some 50% between the ages of 20 and 80 years. Vital capacity diminishes by 25% over the same period as the chest becomes stiffer. Indices of forced expiratory airflow (peak expiratory flow rate, MEF_{50} and FEV_1) show a substantial decline with age. FEV_1 in particular shows a decline of 30 ml per annum (Muiesan *et al.*, 1971). A major factor in the decline of these indices is the reduction in elastic recoil already mentioned.

The resting tidal volume remains constant but dead space ventilation is increased. This slightly less efficient basal ventilation remains adequate because of the diminution of oxygen requirements with age. Arterial pO_2 decreases by about 0.32 mmHg per annum (Mays, 1974)—a drop of almost 20% between the ages of 20 and 80. This change parallels almost exactly the change in elastic recoil throughout life. Arterial pCO_2 remains constant. Oxygen saturation declines by only some 2%. The decrease in pO_2 is thought to be due to two main changes: a decreased transfer factor (diffusing capacity) (Cohn *et al.*, 1954) and increased ventilation–perfusion mismatching. These changes are compounded by the age-related reduction in cardiac output and mixed venous oxygen content. When poorly oxygenated blood circulates through poorly ventilated lung tissue the deleterious effect of ventilation–perfusion mismatch on the arterial pO_2 is increased.

Maximum oxygen uptake during exercise declines by some 50%. Also there is increasing evidence (Kronkenberg and Drage, 1973) that the physiological response to hypoxia and hypercapnia diminishes with age. This is important in clinical practice as the elderly are the group most likely to have chronic respiratory disease, but are also the group least able to respond vigorously to changes in arterial oxygen or carbon dioxide levels. Cellular immunity in the respiratory tract also declines with age (Weksler and Hütteroth, 1974).

NORMAL PLASMA CONSTITUENTS

Given the degree of uncertainty in many aspects of ageing it is hardly surprising that the findings regarding 'normal' blood constituents are far from clear. These constituents have been studied for many years. Early assay techniques were imprecise and quality control poor. In 1964 Woodford-Williams *et al.* surveyed in detail the changes in protein patterns both in normal ageing and in pathology. They established normal base-lines and evaluated the effects of dietary habit, sex, mobility, and pathology. Their results were sometimes quite surprising. They found that over the age of 60 years there was a decrease in the serum albumin. An increase in the total globulin and in the globulin subgroups gave a shift in the albumin/globulin ratio although the total protein remained constant or decreased only slightly. No sex differences were noted. The albumin/globulin ratio declined from a mean of 1.32 (40.4/30.6 in g/l) at age 23 years to 0.87 (32.6/37.6 in g/l) at age 79 years. These findings have been confirmed by several other studies (Calloway *et al.*, 1965; Wallace *et al.*, 1976). This observation is important because a low serum albumin produces a decrease in drug–protein binding—an important factor in drug reactions (Wallace *et al.*, 1976).

It was hardly surprising that Woodford–Williams *et al.* (1964) found that the illest patients had the most abnormal protein patterns. However, this observation proved to be less straightforward than at first sight. On further analysis physical immobility rather than actual disease seemed to be the most important factor, giving the best correlation with albumin decrease and rise in α_2- and γ-globulin changes. No obvious correlation was seen with β-globulin changes. Similar weaker correlations were seen with advancing age, mainly due to its association with decreasing physical mobility.

Surprisingly the quality of nutrition was not associated with hypoalbuminaemia. This conflicts with the often-postulated role of poor dietary intake in causing low serum albumin levels, though doubtless gross malnutrition can cause this effect.

On studying the influence of chronic diseases, renal disease appeared to produce the most profound effect on the serum proteins. The young can produce large γ-globulin increases in chronic disease but the elderly cannot do this. Covariant analysis again suggested that this was due to decreased mobility rather than the disease process.

More recently it has been postulated that the globulin rise is merely due to haemoconcentration following a reduction in the plasma volume with age. A further theory is that the increasingly catabolic state in the elderly decreases albumin synthesis and thus haemoconcentration simply produces a globulin rise to maintain osmotic pressure. While these theories are attractive the evidence to support them is inconclusive.

In a comprehensive study Leask *et al.* (1973) established norms for sixteen blood biochemical parameters in an elderly population in Glasgow, in order that pathological results can be appreciated more precisely. Their results are summarized in Table 1.3. No age-related changes were found in serum sodium, potassium, chloride, bicarbonate, magnesium, and phosphate. On the other hand, serum calcium fell slightly with age; more in men than women. In several studies alkaline phosphatase has been shown to increase with age; more in women than in men. Subclinical vitamin D deficiency has been suggested as an explanation for this finding (McLennan *et al.*, 1972).

There is also a well-documented sex difference and age-related increase in serum urea and creatinine (Ascher and Abernethy, 1970; Milne and Williamson, 1972). Similarly uric acid shows a sex difference and an age-related increase (Reed *et al.*, 1972).

With age there is also some alteration in some of the haemotological indices. Normal values for haemoglobin are essentially unchanged in the elderly (Chalmers *et al.*, 1968). The other indices (PCV, MCH, MCHC, and MCV) are also unchanged with advancing years.

Even in the presence of normal iron stores the serum iron shows a marked age-related decline (Bothwell and Finch, 1962). In the elderly, iron-binding saturation (Se Fe/TIBC %) is probably the most reliable value as levels of 16% or less are rarely found except in iron deficiency (Mitchell and Pegrum, 1971).

Considerable difficulty can occur in the interpretation of serum folate levels in elderly subjects. Values in the region of 1.5 ng/ml are not infrequently found in apparently healthy individuals (Powell and Thomas, 1971). Similar difficulties in interpretation exist with vitamin B12. Estimations of 140 pg/ml should in practice be regarded as the lower limit of normal.

With age there is a decline in the total white cell count due primarily to a reduction in the number of lymphocytes. In the elderly the values for the upper and lower limits of the total white cell count (9000/mm^3 and 3000/mm^3) are different from the normal value in younger subjects (Andrews *et al.*, 1972). This can be of considerable clinical significance.

Table 1.3   'Normal' blood biochemistry in the elderly

Parameter	Change with age	Reference
Sodium	Unchanged	Leask *et al.*, 1973; Roberts, 1959
Chloride	Unchanged	Leask *et al.*, 1973; Wotton and King, 1953
Potassium	Unchanged	Leask *et al.*, 1973; Wotton and King, 1953
Bicarbonate	Unchanged	Leask *et al.*, 1973
Magnesium	Unchanged	Leask *et al.*, 1973
Phosphate	Unchanged	Leask *et al.*, 1973
Calcium	Decreased	Leask *et al.*, 1973
Alkaline phosphatase	Normal (or elevated)	McLennan *et al.*, 1972; (Leask *et al.*, 1973)
Urea	Increased	Milne and Williamson, 1972
Creatinine	Increased	Milne and Williamson, 1972
Uric acid	Increased	Reed *et al.*, 1972
Total protein	Normal/slight decrease	Woodford-Williams, 1964
Serum albumin	Decreased	Woodford-Williams, 1964
Cholestrol	Slight decrease over 75 years (*but still higher than in young*)	Leask *et al.*, 1973; Reed *et al.*, 1972
Bilirubin	Unchanged	Leask *et al.*, 1973

The erythrocyte sedimentation rate rises with age, this change being more marked in women than in men (Bottiger and Svedberg, 1967).

Table 1.4 gives suggested normal values for some commonly measured parameters in the elderly.

Table 1.4   Suggested normal values in the elderly

Constituent	Range
Sodium	135–146 mmol/l
Potassium	3.6–5.2 mmol/l
Chloride	96–108 mmol/l
Bicarbonate	19–31 mmol/l
Total protein	6.1–8.1 g/100 ml (61–81 g/l)
Albumin	3.3–4.9 g/100 ml (33–49 g/l)
Globulin	2.1–4.1 g/100 ml (21–41 g/l)
Phosphate	2.1–4.6 mg/100 ml (0.8–1.3 mmol/l)
Bilirubin	0.3–1.5 mg/100 ml (3–15 μmol/l)
Haemoglobin	12 g/100 ml
Total white cell count	3000/mm^3–9000/mm^3
Urea	22–60 mg/100 ml (2.5–7.5 mmol/l)
Creatinine	0.4–1.9 mg/100 ml (55–125 μmol/l)
Cholesterol	
Female	180–435 mg/100 ml ⎫ (3.1–7.7 mmol/l)
Male	160–345 mg/100 ml ⎭
Calcium	
Female	8.7–10.7 mg/100 ml ⎫ (2.25–2.75 μmol/l)
Male	8.5–10.5 mg/100 ml ⎭
Uric acid	
Female	2.1–7.7 mg/100 ml. (0.12–0.33 mmol/l)
Male	3.1–7.9 mg/100 ml. (0.12–0.39 mmol/l)
Alkaline phosphatase (K-A units)	5–20 (35–115 i.u./l)

REFERENCES AND BIBLIOGRAPHY

Addis, T. (1948) *Glomerular nephritis, Diagnosis and Treatment.* Macmillan, New York.

Adler, S. *et al.* (1968) Effect of acute loading on urinary acid excretion by the ageing human kidney. *J. Lab. Clin. Med.*, **72**, 278.

Andrews, G. R. *et al.* (1972) The leucocyte count in old age. *Age and Ageing*, **1**, 239.

Ascher, A. W. and Abernethy, M. (1970) Clinical significance of dysuria in women. *Brit. Med. J.*, **2**, 754.

Bender, J. (1964) Pharmacological aspects of ageing. *J. Am. Geriat. Soc.*, **12**, 114.

Bender, J. (1968) Effect of age on intestinal absorption. *J. Am. Geriat. Soc.*, **16**, 1331.

Bothwell, T. H. and Finch, C. A. (1962) *Iron Metabolism*. Little, Brown & Co., Boston.

Bottiger, L. E. and Svedberg, C. A. (1967) Normal erythrocyte sedimentation rate and age. *BMJ*, **2**, 85.

Brandfonbrener, M., Landowne, M., and Shock, N. W. (1955) Changes in cardiac output with age. *Circulation*, **12**, 577.

Calloway, N. O. and Merrill, R. S. (1965) Bromsulphthalein clearance and bilirubin. *J. Am. Geriat. Soc.*, **13**, 594.

Calloway, N. O., Foley, C. F., and Lagerbloom, P. (1965) Uncertainties in geriatric data: organ size. *J. Am. Geriat. Soc.*, **13**, 20.

Carr, R. D., Smith, M. J., and Keil, P. G. (1960) The liver in the ageing process. *Arch. Path.*, **70**, 1.

Castleden, C. M. *et al.* (1975) The effects of age on plasma levels of practolol and propranolol. *Br. J. Clin. Pharmacol.*, **2**, 303.

Chalmers, D. G. *et al.* (1968) The haemoglobin level of fit elderly people. *Lancet*, **2**, 261.

Cockcroft, D. W. and Gault, M. H. (1976) Prediction of creatinine clearance from serum creatinine. *Nephron*, **16**, 31–41.

Cohn, J. E. *et al.* (1954) Max. diffusing capacity of the lung in normal male subjects of different ages. *J. Appl. Physiol.*, **6**, 588.

Cohn, J. E. and Donoso, H. D. (1963) Mechanical properties of the lung in normal men over 60 years. *J. Clin. Invest.*, **42**, 1406.

Cook, C. D., Mead, J., and Orzalesi, M. M. (1964) Static volume–pressure characteristics of the respiratory system during maximal effort. *J. Appl. Physiol.*, **19**, 1016–22.

Corsellis, J. A. N. (1976) Ageing and the dementias. In W. Blackwood and J. A. N. Corsellis (eds), *Greenfields Neuropathology*, pp. 796–848. Arnold, London.

Cottrell, L. (1940) Histological variation with age in normal nerve trunks. *Arch. Neurol. Psychiat.*, **43**, 1138.

Davies, D. F. and Shock, N. W. (1950) Age changes in glomerular filtration rate, effective renal plasma flow and tubular excretory capacity in adult males. *J. Clin. Invest.*, **29**, 496.

Davison, A. N. (1978) Biochemical aspects of the ageing brain. *Age and Ageing*, **7** (suppl. 4).

Edelman, L. S. and Leibman, J. (1959) Anatomy of body water and electrolytes. *Am. J. Med.*, **27**, 256–77.

Evans, D. A. P., Manley, K. A., and McKusick, V. A. (1960) Genetic control of isoniazid metabolism in man. *Brit. Med. J.*, **42**, 485.

Farah, F. *et al.* (1977) Hepatic drug acetylation and oxidation: effects of ageing in man. *Brit. Med. J.*, **2**, 155–6.

Fazekas, J. F., Klen, J., and Finnerty, F. A. (1955) Influence of age and vascular disease on cerebral haemodynamics and metabolism. *Am. J. Med.*, **18**, 477.

Flood, C. *et al.* (1967) The metabolism and excretion of aldosterone in elderly subjects. *J. Clin. Invest.*, **46**, 960.

Forbes, G. R. and Reina, J. C. (1970) Adult lean body mass declines with age: some longitudinal observations. *Metabolism*, **19**, 653–63.

Freston, J. W. and Englert, E. (1967) The effect of age and excessive body weight on the distribution and metabolism of bromsulphthalein. *Clin. Sci.*, **33**, 301–12.

Geokas, M. C. and Haverback, B. J. (1969) The ageing gastro-intestinal tract. *Am. J. Surg.*, **117**, 881.

Goldman, R. (1971) Decline in organ function with age. In I. Rossman (ed.), *Clinical Geriatrics*. Lippincott, Philadelphia.

Goldring, W. and Chasis, H. (1944) *Hypertension and Hypertensive Disease*, p. 56. Commonwealth Fund, New York.

Gramath, A., Jonsson, B., and Strandell, T. (1964) Circulation in healthy old men, studied by right heart catheterisation at rest and exercise in supine and sitting position. *Acta Med. Scand.*, **176**, 425.

Gregerman, R. I. (1967) In Williams (ed.), *Endocrines in Ageing*. Charles C. Thomas, Springfield.

Gregerman, R. I. and Solomon, N. (1967) The thyroid in stress. *J. Clin. Endocrinol.*, **27**, 93.

Gregerman, R. I., Gaffney, G. W., and Shock, N. W. (1962) Thyroxine turnover in euthyroid man with special reference to changes with age. *J. Clin. Invest.*, **41**, 2065–74.

Harris, R. (1970) *The Management of Geriatric Cardiovascular Disease*. J. B. Lippincott Co., Philadelphia.

John, R. and Thomas, J. (1972) Chemical composition of elastins isolated from aortas and pulmonary tissues of humans of different ages. *Biochem. J.*, **127**, 261–9.

Kampmann, J. P., Sindling, J., and Møller-Jørgensen, I. (1975) Effect of age on liver function. *Geriatrics*, **30**, 91–5.

Kendall, M. J. (1970) The influence of age on the xylose absorption rest. *Gut*, **11**, 498.

Kronkenberg, R. S. and Drage, C. W. (1973) Attenuation of the ventilatory and heart rate responses to hypoxia and hypercapnia with ageing in normal men. *J. Clin. Invest.*, **52**, 1812–79.

Landowne, M. *et al.* (1955) The relation of age to certain measures of the performance of heart and circulation. *Circulation*, **11**, 567.

Landowne, M. and Stanley, J. (1960) *Ageing of the Cardiovascular System*. Am. Assoc. Adv. Sci., Washington, DC.

Leask, R. G. S., Andrews, G. R., and Caird, F. I. (1973) Normal values for sixteen blood constituents in the elderly. *Age and Ageing*, **2**, 14.

Lesser, G. T., Kumar, I., and Steele, J. M. (1963) Changes in body composition with age. *Ann. NY Acad. Sci.*, **110**, 578.

McLennan, W. J., Caird, F. I., and Macleod, C. (1972) Diet and bone rarefaction in old age. *Age and Ageing*, **1**, 131.

Master, A. M. and Lasser, R. P. (1961) Blood pressure elevation in the elderly. In A. N. Brest and J. H. Moyer (eds), *Hypertension: Recent Advances*. Lea & Febiger, Philadelphia.

Mays, E. E. (1974) Unpublished observations.

Meyer, J. and Nechles, H. (1940) Enzyme secretion. *JAMA*, **115**, 2050.

Meyer, J. *et al.* (1943) Studies in old age. VII. *J. Gastroenterol.*, **1**, 876.

Miller, J. H. *et al.* (1953) Age differences in renal tubular response to ADH. *J. Gerontol.*, **8**, 446.

Miller, J. H., McDonald, R. K., and Shock, N. W. (1951) The renal excretion of p-aminohippurate in the aged individual. *J. Gerontol.*, **6**, 413.

Miller, J. H., McDonald, R. K., and Shock, N. W. (1952) Age changes in the maximal rate of renal tubular reabsorption of glucose. *J. Gerontol.*, **7**, 196.

16

Milne, J. S. and Williamson, J. (1972) Plasma urea concentration in older people. *Gerontol. Clin.*, **14**, 32.

Mitchell, T. R. and Pegrum, G. D. (1971) The diagnosis of mild iron deficiency in the elderly. *Gerontol. Clin.*, **13**, 296.

Mittman, C. *et al.* (1965) Relationship between chest wall and pulmonary compliance and age. *J. Appl. Physiol.*, **20**, 1211–16.

Moller, E., McIntosh, J. F., and Van Slyke, D. D. (1928) Studies of urea excretion. II. *J. Clin. Invest.*, **6**, 427–65.

Montoye, J., Willis, P. W. III, and Cunningham, D. A. (1968) Heart rate response to submaximal exercise: relation to age and sex. *J. Gerontol.*, **23**, 27.

Moore, F. *et al.* (1963) *The Body Cell Mass and its Supporting Environment.* W. B. Saunders, Philadelphia.

Muiesan, G., Sorbini, C. A., and Grassi, V. (1971) Respiratory function in the aged. *Bull. Physiopathol. Resp.*, **7**, 973–1009.

Pierce, J. A. (1963) Age related changes in the fibrous proteins in the lungs. *Arch. Environ. Health*, **6**, 50–4.

Powell, D. E. B. and Thomas, J. H. (1971) *Blood Disorders in the Elderly.* Wright, Bristol.

Reed, A. H. *et al.* (1972) Estimation of normal ranges from a controlled sample survey. Sex and age related influences on the tests. *Clin. Chem.*, **18**, 57.

Ritschel, W. A. (1976) Pharmacokinetic approach to drug dosing in the aged. *J. Am. Geriat. Soc.*, **24**, 344.

Roberts, L. B. (1967) The normal ranges, with statistical analysis, for seventeen blood constituents. *Clin. Chim. Acta*, **16**, 69.

Roessle, R. and Roulet, F. (1932) *Mass und Zahl in der Pathologie.* J. Springer, Berlin.

Salem, S. A. M. *et al.* (1978) Reduced induction of drug metabolism in the elderly. *Age and Ageing*, **7**, 68–73.

Sapp, O. L. *et al.* (1964) Effect of ageing on intestinal absorption of sugars. *Clin. Res.*, **12**, 31.

Sherlock, S. *et al.* (1950) Splanchnic blood flow in man by B.S.P. method: relation of peripheral plasma B.S.P. to calc. blood flow. *J. Lab. Clin. Med.*, **35**, 923.

Shock, N. W. (1952) Age changes in renal function. In *Cowdrey's Problems of Ageing*, pp. 614–30. Williams & Wilkins, Baltimore.

Shock, N. W. *et al.* (1963) Age change in body water and its relationship to basal oxygen consumption in males. *J. Gerontol.*, **8**, 388 (Abstr.).

Thompson, E. N. and Williams, R. (1965) Effect of age on liver function with reference to bromsulphthalein excretion. *Gut*, **6**, 266.

Van Pilsum, J. F. and Seljeskog, E. L. (1958) Long term endogenous creatinine clearance in man. *Proc. Soc. Exp. Biol. (NY)*, **97**, 270–2.

Wallace, S., Whiting, B., and Runcie, J. (1976) Factors affecting drug binding in plasma of elderly patients. *Brit. J. Clin. Pharmacol.*, **3**, 327–30.

Warren, P. M. (1978) Age changes in small intestinal mucosa. *Lancet* (ii), 849(c).

Weksler, M. E. and Hütteroth, T. H. (1974) Impaired lympocyte function in aged humans. *J. Clin. Invest.*, **53**, 99–104.

Whittaker, J. A. and Evans, D. A. P. (1970) Genetic control of phenylbutazone metabolism in man, *BMJ*, **4**, 323.

Woodford-Williams, E. *et al.* (1964) Serum protein patterns in normal and pathological ageing. *Gerontol. Clin.*, **10**, 86.

Wotton, I. D. P. and King, E. J. (1953) Normal values for blood constituents: interhospital differences. *Lancet*, i, 470.

Wright, R. R. (1961) Elastic tissue of normal and emphysematous lungs. A tridimensional histological study. *Am. J. Pathol.*, **39**, 355–67.

Chapter 2

Age and drug handling

Before considering the prescribing of drugs in various diseases, we need first to examine the steps by which the body handles drugs—namely absorption, distribution, metabolism, and excretion—and how these processes are influenced by the physiological and anatomical changes detailed in Chapter One.

ABSORPTION

Most drugs are taken orally, so attention will be focused on absorption from the gastrointestinal tract with a brief comment of parenteral administration. Two main aspects are important in drug absorption: the physicochemiocal properties of the drug and individual subjects' idiosyncracies (Table 2.1).

Drug formulation is highly important. If the taste or size of tablet is too deterring then the medicine will be taken erratically, if at all. The drug itself may be unstable unless mixed at the last minute, kept at a specific temperature, stored out of the light, etc. Fortunately, advances in the pharmaceutical industry have made these factors much less important. The prime physicochemical factors governing drug absorption are:

(1) the drug's degree of lipid solubility—high lipid solubility is essential to ensure good passive diffusion across the cell membrane;
(2) the degree of ionization; only unionized forms are able to cross the cell membranes freely—ionization is influenced by pH, as will be discussed later;
(3) the size of the molecule is vital.

Drugs are only absorbed in aqueous solution, so if the drug is to be given in solid form (as a tablet or a powder) then distintegration and dissolution rates becomes important. The dissolution rate can be greatly influenced by the formulation of the preparation or the particular drug salt chosen (BP policy on dissolution testing, 1978). Minor changes in bioavailability can lead to major toxicity problems when using drugs with narrow therapeutic margins such a digoxin, phenytoin, warfarin, or lithium.

18

Drug absorption can be slowed down by using enteric-coated or sustained-release formulations. These preparations are normally substantially more expensive than ordinary tablets, and in some cases their usefulness is uncertain. Some drugs are specially formulated to avoid absorption; for example, the prodrug sulphasalazine is not absorbed in the upper gastrointestinal tract but colonic bacteria split it into 5-aminosalicyclate and sulphapyrazine.

Absorption from the gut into the blood stream is achieved by four main methods: passive diffusion, active transport, pinocytosis, and filtration through pores. Passive diffusion is by far the most important method for drug absorption, but the other three methods will be first considered briefly for completeness.

Active transport uses energy to form a complex which passes through the membrane, releasing the drug into the blood stream. This highly specific method of absorption is chiefly for amino acids and vitamins. Drug absorption by this method is unusual unless drugs are very closely related to a naturally occurring substance, e.g. methyldopa. This form of absorption can be saturated and blocked. Pinocytosis is unimportant apart from the very few macromolecules absorbed into the lymphatics. Filtration through tissue pores is limited to very small molecules

Table 2.1 Factors influencing drug absorption

Physiocochemical properties of the individual drug
    Molecular sizc
    Lipid–water partition coefficient
    Degree of ionization
    Formulation
    Metabolism by intestinal bacteria and/or enzymes
    Similarity to naturally occurring substances

Characteristics of the individual patient
    Compliance with therapeutic regimen
    pH of the gastrointestinal tract
    Rate of gastric emptying
    Intestinal motility
    Absorptive surface area of the small bowel
    Splanchnic and hepatic blood flow
    Gastrointestinal disease
    Presence of disease such as congestive cardiac failure

Other factors
    Large meal
    High fluid intake
    Drug interactions

(molecular weight below 100) which can be either lipophilic or hydrophilic. The total pore area is very small (Binns, 1971).

Passive diffusion is the main method of drug absorption. It cannot be saturated. Structurally similar drugs are transferred independently and there is no cross-interference. The process involves no energy expenditure. The drug must first be present at the cell membrane in aqueous solution. It then dissolves into the lipid membrane and passes out the other side again into the aqueous phase. The rate of transfer across the membrane is proportional to the concentration gradient and to the lipid–water partition coefficient: the higher the coefficient, the faster the absorption. Most drugs are weak acids or bases, so occur in both ionized and unionized forms. The proportion of each form depends on the pH and they are equal at pK_a (the negative log of the acidic dissociation constant). If the pH is increased, acidic drugs ionize more, and basic drugs less. Ionized forms are not very lipid-soluble and hence do not permeate cell membranes well; so pH greatly influences the rate of transfer. This is the basis of Brodie's (1964) pH partition theory and explains why some drugs are not absorbed at all: for instance, streptomycin is completely ionized and sulphaguanidine is not lipid-soluble. However, this excellent work was carried out in rats using drugs in solution. This may explain some of the discrepancies found between Brodie's results and clinical practice. Acidic drugs such as aspirin, warfarin, or phenobarbitone will be at their most unionized in the acidic medium of the stomach and hence at their most permeable and easily absorbed. But in fact gastric absorption is slow—absorption is better in the relative neutrality of the upper small intestine. This is thought to be due to the vastly greater intestinal surface area. In the elderly there is also a rise in gastric pH: this has been shown to increase the rate of gastric emptying (Richey and Bender, 1977). The rate of paracetamol absorption appears to reflect exactly the rate of gastric emptying (Prescott, 1974). It has long been assumed that the upper small intestine is the site of maximum absorption. This is highly logical. Even after a slight age-related decline the absorptive surface area is still about the size of two full-sized tennis courts. It is also here that the maximum drug concentrations are reached, increasing the concentration gradient to speed up passive diffusion.

In 1964 Bender found quite considerable decreases in the absorption of various food substances in the elderly. However, most of these substances are absorbed by specific active transport mechanisms so a straightforward correlation to drug absorption cannot be made. In an excellent study using propicillin (Simon *et al.*, 1972) no age alteration in

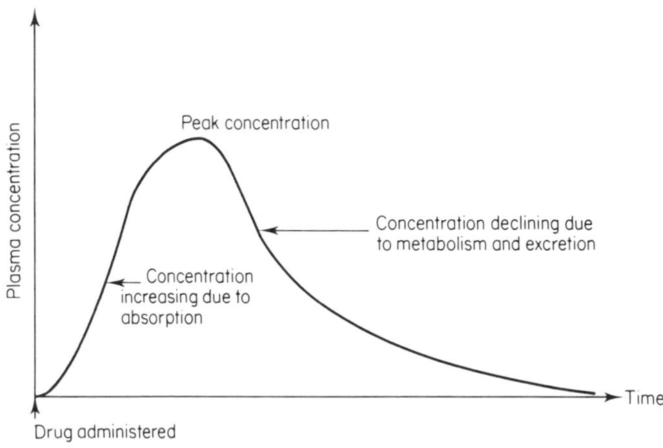

Fig. 2.1   Typical time course–concentration pattern for drug absorption

absorption rate was found. Some other studies in this field give slightly dubious results because they used highly refined solutions prepared specifically by the pharmaceutical company rather than commercial preparations. In several excellent studies no alteration has been found in the absorption of paracetamol, sulphamethiazole (Triggs *et al.*, 1975), tetracycline (Kramer *et al.*, 1978), aspirin and practolol (Castleden *et al.*, 1977a), theophylline (Cussack *et al.*, 1979) with age.

Nevertheless altered gastric and intestinal motility have been postulated as important factors in drug absorption in the elderly. Alterations in the rate of gastric emptying affect the rate rather than the extent of drug absorption. The rate of absorption is only important where an immediate effect is required, e.g. analgesics, hypnotics or (to a lesser extent) antibiotics. Absorption rate is not important where drugs are taken chronically since the steady-state concentrations are not affected. An excellent example is digoxin, where there is a substantial age-related delay in absorption but total uptake is not significantly affected (76% absorbed at age 70 and 84% absorbed at age 40) (Cussack *et al.*, 1979).

Drugs which themselves alter gastroinestinal motility can alter the uptake patterns of other drugs. For instance, the uptake rate of digoxin is increased by propantheline and decreased by metoclopramide. However, the digoxin preparations used in these studies were old-fashioned slow-release formulations: this effect is not seen with the new standard (Lanoxin) formulation. Other drugs whose absorption can be significantly influenced in this way are listed in Table 2.2.

Table 2.2 Drug–drug interactions influencing absorption

Drug	Drug influencing absorption	Effect	Points to note
Digoxin	Cholestyramine	Decreased digoxin by binding	
Digoxin	Metoclopramide	Decreased digoxin by influencing gut motility	Only with old slow-dissolution digoxin preparations
Digoxin	Propantheline	Increased digoxin by influencing gut motility	
Warfarin	Cholestyramine	Decreased warfarin by binding	
Tetracycline	Antacids	Chelation	If necessary always give at least 2 h apart
Iron	Antacids	Chelation	
Lithium	Metoclopramide	Speeds absorption	Makes monitoring blood levels more difficult
Lithium	Propantheline	Delays absorption	
			Other drugs with atropine-like action produce similar effect (e.g. pheno-thiazines or tricyclic antidepressants)

One important aspect which has received relatively little study is the effect of other intestinal contents on drug absorption. Enzymes are secreted into the gastrointestinal tract in vast quantities. Many of these, especially the esterases, have an important role to play in the splitting of drug glucuronides excreted by the liver. The effect of age on this aspect is not known.

The effect of food on the bioavailability of drugs has long been thought to be purely mechanical. However, recent studies have shown that this simplistic view is no longer tenable. The food constituents have been shown to exert both long- and short-term effects on almost every facet of drug absorption and biotransformation. The effects of food vary widely, even for closely related drugs in the same drug family. Food can inflence the disintegration and dissolution of the drug. It also exerts an influence on transit time and metabolic transformation. These effects are of considerable importance as the drugs involved are widely used, e.g. hydrochlorothiazide, metoprolol, antibiotics, etc. The drugs for which evidence of altered bioavailability with food exists are outlined in Table 2.3. The effects are highly individual, and for many commonly used drugs no information exists at this time.

Fluid volume can have a marked effect on drug absorption. Most drugs seem to be better absorbed when taken with a little water. Fluid may stimulate gastric emptying and aid drug dissolution, especially for drugs that are not freely water-soluble.

Disease itself can greatly influence drug absorption. The classic example of this in the elderly is congestive cardiac failure which can delay the absorption of thiazides, digoxin, and quinidine. The mechanism is thought to be due to a reduction in splanchnic blood flow and intestinal mucosal oedema. Diseases causing malabsorption can also reduce drug absorption. Drugs absorbed from specific sites can be very seriously affected, for instance vitamin B12 when the terminal ileum is involved in Crohn's disease, or iron from the duodeum and upper jejunum when enteropathy is present. Biliary obstruction can reduce the absorption of some fat-soluble drugs. These effects are summarized in Table 2.4.

A few drugs that are taken orally are designed to be absorbed directly from the oral mucosa. In theory this method circumvents the portal circulation and gives faster uptake. In practice, however, few drugs given by this method have stood the test of time—the most important survivor being trinitrin.

The rectal route would also in theory bypass the portal circulation. However, the venous anastomoses are highly variable and for cultural reasons in this country the rectal route is distinctly unpopular.

Table 2.3   Influence of food on the bioavailability of drugs

Drug	Effect on bioavailability	Mechanism	Reference
Propranolol	Increased	Reduces hepatic first-pass metabolism	Melander, 1977a
Metoprolol	Increased	Reduces hepatic first-pass metabolism	Melander *et al.*, 1977a
Hydrochloro-thiazide	Increased	Slower gastric emptying aids absorption by slower delivery to uptake site	Beermann and Groschinsky-Grind, 1978
Hydrallazine	Increased	Reduces enzymic metabolism in the liver	Jenne, 1965
Digoxin	Bioavailability unchanged	Rate of absorption decreased; extent of absorption un-changed	Johnson *et al.*, 1978
Theophylline	Unchanged	See Note (1) below	Welling *et al.*, 1975
Isoniazid	Reduced (up to 50%)* (Mitchison, 1973)	Alteration in gastric emptying and pH. Note (2)*	Melander *et al.*, 1976
Rifampicin	Reduced	Absorption reduced	Acocella, 1978
Penicillin Erythromycin (see Note 3)	Reduced	Delayed gastric emptying increases degradation	
Tetracycline	Reduced	Chelates with metallic ions in food	Neuvonen, 1976
Amoxycillin	Unchanged	—	Neu, 1974
Metronidazole	Unchanged	—	Kamme *et al.*, 1978
Nitrofurantoin	Increased	Delayed gastric emptying increases dissolution	Jaffe, 1975
Griseofulvin	Increased	If fatty meal it aids dissolution	Crounse, 1963
Phenytoin	Increased	Increased absorption better tablet dissolution (Note 4)	Melander *et al.*, 1978

Table 2.3   continued

Drug	Effect on bioavailability	Mechanism	Reference
Carbamazepine	Increased	Bile secretion improves dissolution	Levy *et al.*, 1975
Oxazepam	Unchanged	—	Melander *et al.*, 1977b
Diazepam	Increased	By enhancing the enterohepatic recycling	Linnoila *et al.*, 1975
Paracetamol	Reduced (more so in specific circumstances)	If carbohydrate-rich meal due to interaction with pectin.	Jaffe *et al.*, 1971
		Reduced by delayed gastric emptying	Heading *et al.*, 1973
Aspirin	Reduced (varies with the preparation)	Food acting as diluent	Bogentoft *et al.*, 1978
Anticoagulants	Enhanced	Food delays gastric emptying and stimulates bile, thus increasing dissolution	Melander and Wahlin, 1978

Notes:
1. Theophylline—changes in the balance between protein/carbohydrate ratio influence theophylline excretion (Kappas *et al.*, 1976).
2. Isoniazid—can be reduced by antacids (Hurwitz, 1977).
3. Erythromycin stearate—may have enhanced bioavailability with food (Malmborg, 1978).
4. Phenytoin—due to the variability of effect of food patients should be recommended to take their phenytoin at the same time in relation to meals.
* Clinically important.

It has always been expounded that the parenteral route is faster and more reliable. In most instance this is so, but not always. In particular, uptake from intramuscular injections can be poor and unreliable if the peripheral circulation is poor.

DISTRIBUTION

After absorption the distribution of a drug is largely influenced by its polarity, its degree of protein-binding and variations in the individual patient. Lipophilic drugs are widely distributed as they pass easily across

Table 2.4 Disease processes and their effect on drug handling

Pathology	Drug involved	Effect	Reference
Pyloric stenosis	Aspirin	Absorption impaired	Heading *et al.*, 1973
	Paracetamol	Absorption impaired	Nimmo *et al.*, 1973
Slow intestinal transit	Chlorpromazine	Increased metabolism in the gut wall	Rivera-Calimlin *et al.*, 1978
Coeliac disease (effect inconsistent)	Penicillin V	Decreased absorption	Parsons *et al.*, 1977
	Thyroxine	Decreased absorption	Parsons *et al.*, 1977
	Propranolol	Increased absorption	Parsons *et al.*, 1977
	Cotrimoxazole	Increased absorption	Parsons *et al.*, 1977
Crohn's disease (effect inconsistent)	Lincomycin	Decreased absorption	Parsons *et al.*, 1977
	Metronidazole	Slightly reduced absorption	Parsons *et al.*, 1977
	Cotrimoxazole	Increased absorption	Parsons *et al.*, 1977
Liver disease (effects highly variable)	Albumin binding metabolism	Requires detailed knowledge of metabolic pathways (see Chapter 8)	
Acute myocardial infarction	Procainamide	Oral absorption decreased (especially if narcotic analgesics also given)	
Congestive cardiac failure	Lignocaine	Toxicity due to excretion	Odutola *et al.*, 1978
	Phenylbutazone Carbenoxalone	Precipitate congestive cardiac failure due to mineralocorticoid activity	Odutola *et al.*, 1978
Uraemia	Cloxacillin Chlorpropamide Pindolol	Decreased absorption	Fabre and Balant, 1976

More detailed consideration of the effect of renal impairment will be made in Chapter 10.

the membranes and accumulate in the fat tissues. Polar drugs are, however, confined to extracellular fluids since they do not cross membranes easily. Thus the phospholipid membrane structure is very important in determining distribution patterns. For a lipid-soluble drug the rate of membrane transport, and hence rate of distribution, is also influenced by tissue differences in pH and fat content, as well as the amount of tissue protein with a high affinity for that particular drug.

Individual idiosyncracies are magnified by age-related changes in body composition and function, such as change in body proteins, regional blood flow (Rowland *et al.*, 1973), receptor sites and most obviously alterations in body fats and fluid volumes (Brodie, 1964; Klotz, 1976) (Tables 2.5 and 2.6). The end results of the age-related changes in body composition is to alter the apparent volume of distribution of a drug. There is considerable confusion about the exact alterations in pharmacokinetics these changes cause (Mitchard, 1979).

Drugs are transported to their site of action via the circulation, largely bound to plasma proteins and erythrocytes. The chief protein carrier is serum albumin but lipoproteins, α_1-glycoprotein, and some of the globulins also have a role to play. Drug distribution, metabolism, and excretion are not sequential but simultaneous processes; so an alteration in protein binding can also indirectly influence these other mechanisms, and affect the duration and intensity of drug action.

The exterior of a protein is made up chiefly of amino acids with their

Table 2.5 Drugs where protein binding and its relation to age have been studied

Drug	Protein binding change	Reference
Carbenoxolone	Binding decreased	Hayes *et al.*, 1977
Chlormethiazole	Binding decreased	Nation *et al.*, 1977a
Desmethyldiazepam	Binding unchanged	Klotz and Miller-Seyditz, 1979
Diazepam	Binding unchanged	Klotz *et al.*, 1976
Lorazepam	Binding unchanged	Kraus *et al.*, 1978
Penicillin	Binding unchanged	Bender *et al.*, 1975
Pethidine	Binding decreased	Chan *et al.*, 1975
Phenobarbitone	Binding unchanged	Bender *et al.*, 1975
Phenylbutazone	Binding decreased	Wallace *et al.*, 1976
Phenytoin	Binding decreased/ unchanged	Hayes *et al.*, 1975b; Bender *et al.*, 1975
Quinidine	Binding unchanged	Ochs *et al.*, 1978
Salicylate	Binding unchanged	Wallace *et al.*, 1976
Tolbutamide	Binding decreased	Miller *et al.*, 1977
Warfarin	Binding decreased/ unchanged	Hayes *et al.*, 1975a; Shepherd *et al.*, 1978

Table 2.6 Drugs where volume of distribution (V_d) has been studied in relation to age

Drug	Change in V_d	Reference
Chlordiazepoxide	Increased/decreased	Klotz *et al.*, 1975; Shader *et al.*, 1977
Chlormethiazole	Increased	Nation *et al.*, 1976
Desmethyldiazepam	Unchanged	Klotz and Miller-Seyditz, 1979
Diazepam	Increased	Klotz *et al.*, 1975
Digoxin	Unchanged/decreased	Cusack *et al.*, 1979; Ewy *et al.*, 1969
Ethanol	Decreased	Vestal *et al.*, 1977
Lignocaine	Increased	Nation *et al.*, 1977b
Lorazepam	Unchanged	Kraus *et al.*, 1978
Oxazepam	Unchanged	Shull *et al.*, 1976
Paracetamol	Unchanged	Triggs *et al.*, 1975
Phenazone	Decreased	O'Malley *et al.*, 1971
Phenylbutazone	Unchanged/increased	Triggs, 1975; O'Malley *et al.*, 1971
Propicillin	Decreased	Simon *et al.*, 1972
Qunidine	Unchanged	Ochs *et al.*, 1978
Theophylline	Unchanged	Cusack *et al.*, 1980
Tolbutamide	Increased	Miller *et al.*, 1977

projecting side-chains. Any given protein may have several specific structures and reactive groups which allow the reversible binding of several different-shaped molecules. The binding may involve ionic, hydrogen, hydrophobic, or van der Waals bonds. Small molecules can even enter the protein via pores. Once the molecule has attached to the protein carrier it circulates through the body until it dissociates and bonds with another macromolecule.

Serum albumin (molecular weight = 66,400) exists in several closely related configurations. On each type the number and position of the binding sites for different drugs may vary. Albumin has a high affinity for acidic drugs such as acetylsalicyclic acid, warfarin, phenylbutazone, penicillins, or sulphonamides. To date two separate binding sites have been described on albumin.

Site I is the less specific of the two sites. It can bind a range of structurally unrelated drugs, e.g. warfarin, phenylbutazone, phenytoin, sodium valproate, and many sulphonamides. Warfarin binding at this site seems to be specific and warfarin displacement by other drugs has been used to identify their binding site as site I.

Site II appears to be more specific and the site marker here is diazepam.

Some site II drugs, e.g. ibuprofen and its analogues, also have a slight affinity for site I. In addition to drugs plasma proteins also bind a range of endogenous substances such as bilirubin, L-tryptophan, vitamins, and fatty acids. Bilirubin and fatty acids have their own specific binding sites on serum albumin. High concentrations of free fatty acids (e.g. during heparin infusion) can influence drug binding (Storstein, 1976; Nilsen *et al.*, 1977). However, normal physiological variations in free fatty acids usually have little influence on drug binding.

Acidic and basic drugs tend to bind to different proteins. Albumin has a high affinity for acidic drugs while basic lipophilic drugs tend to be bound to α_1-acid glycoproteins and the lipoproteins (Borga *et al.*, 1977; Fremstad *et al.*, 1976). The latter group include propranolol, alprenolol, chlorpromazine, imipramine, and quinidine.

The law of mass action governs the reversible drug–protein relationship. The rate of dissociation of the drug–protein complex is extremely rapid ($T_{1/2}$ approximately 20 milliseconds). Since the perfusion time of an organ is greater than this, complex dissociation is not a rate-limiting factor in drug uptake by body organs. To cross cell membranes a drug must be in the free unbound form. The drug-protein complex is therefore a drug reservoir; as free drug crosses into cells, more drug–protein complex dissociates. The free unionized drug is considered to be the pharmacologically active form. The controlling factor for drug distribution into the tissues will thus be the concentration of this free unionized form. This in turn is governed by the total concentration of the drug, the serum level of the protein carrier, and the proportion of the total drug bound to protein. The avidity of protein binding is determined by two binding constants—the number of binding sites and the apparent association constant.

Drugs vary widely in their binding power to tissue proteins. Highly tissue-bound drugs can be cleared completely from the plasma during one passage through an organ. For instance, virtually all propranolol, bound or free, is cleared from the blood by one passage through the liver. Here binding to plasma proteins does not hinder rapid tissue uptake: binding merely increases the total drug available for uptake from the serum.

Increasing age will affect this basic pharmacology in several ways. In chronic administration body size will influence drug levels; the larger the subject the lower the serum or tissue level for a given dose. During ageing one tends to lose height and weight. This diminution will tend to increase drug levels. Also, as mentioned earlier, ageing diminishes lean body mass and increases body fat. So polar drugs highly bound to tissue proteins will have smaller distribution volumes and elevated plasma concentrations in the elderly. An elegant study on the highly polar drug digoxin (Ewy *et al.*, 1969) shows this effect beautifully. This and similar studies are detailed in Table 2.6. In contrast, lipid-soluble drugs will have larger tissue reservoirs and longer apparent half-lives in the elderly.

Thus distribution changes in the elderly can be summarized as an increase in V_d (distribution volume) and a decrease in blood levels for lipid-soluble drugs, while for polar drugs V_d decreases and blood levels rise. In simpler terms, in old age polar drugs are distributed less widely and non-polar drugs more widely.

The serum albumin also declines with age. This decline may be aggravated by immobility and chronic disease (Woodford-Williams *et al.*, 1964). The effect of the changes in protein binding on pharmacokinetics has been reviewed in an excellent paper by Jusko and Gretch (1977). Several drugs, such as phenytoin, pethidine, and phenylbutazone, have been shown to have reduced protein binding in the elderly. The decline in binding seems to be related to the serum albumin level (Wallace *et al.*, 1976). The binding of salicylate, phenylbutazone, and sulphadiazine has been shown to be reduced in the elderly. Hayes *et al.* (1975b) and Hooper *et al.* (1974) showed that low serum albumin can increase the free level of phenytoin. This was contested by Bender *et al.* (1975). A correlation has been shown between mean daily prednisone dosage, serum albumin level and the incidence of side-effects (Lewis *et al.*, 1971). Side-effects were twice as likely to occur when the serum albumin was below 25 g/l. Hypoalbuminaemia increased the levels of free prednisolone, the chief metabolite. Prednisolone was 65% bound when the albumin was 40 g/l but only 48% bound when the albumin was 25 g/l.

This reduced binding means that drugs are more easily displaced from binding sites by competitors, giving greater increases in free plasma concentrations (Wallace *et al.*, 1976). Polypharmacy could be more dangerous in the elderly (as well as being more common). In practice the incidence of toxic reactions rises markedly with the number of drugs taken (Smith *et al.*, 1966). Not surprisingly, toxic reactions are indeed much more common in old age (Smith *et al.*, 1966).

Changes in protein binding have important effects only when the drug is highly protein-bound. If only a small proportion of the drug is protein-bound, quite major changes in protein binding have little effect on distribution. The drug's volume of distribution (V_d) is the volume required to contain the total body drugs were it at the concentration found in the plasma. This volume of distribution modifies the effect of plasma protein binding changes. In strongly tissue-bound drugs with a high V_d, only a small fraction of the drug will be bound to plasma protein; so changes in

Table 2.7   Parameters of distribution which influence drug
handling in the aged

Volume of distribution	Erythrocyte binding
Protein binding	Urine concentration

plasma protein binding will have relatively little effect on overall distribution. Conversely, for drugs like warfarin with a low V_d, there is little or no 'tissue reservoir' to cushion changes in the plasma protein binding; so small changes in plasma protein binding can substantially affect serum drug levels.

Erythrocyte binding of drugs can sometimes be important in the total distribution. One study contrasted the binding of pethidine to erythrocytes in the young (below 30 years) and the old (above 70 years) (Chan *et al.*, 1975). It found significantly more pethidine bound to erythrocytes in the young. Haematocrits and erythrocyte protein structure were the same in the two groups. The study concluded that the difference in erythrocyte binding was sufficient to account for the plasma pethidine levels in the elderly being twice as high as in the young. This negative correlation of binding and age was verified by Mather *et al.* (1975). Similar age-related changes in red cell binding have been found for chlormethiazole (Nation *et al.*, 1977). Table 2.7 summarizes the parameters of distribution which have produced altered drug handling in the elderly.

METABOLISM

As with other aspects of drug handling, age also affects drug metabolism. As mentioned in Chapter 1, the size of the liver declines with age as does the number of functioning hepatic cells (Sato *et al.*, 1970). The hepatic blood flow declines in parallel with the splanchnic blood flow as the years advance (0.3–1.5% per annum) (Geokas and Haverback, 1969). If bromsulphthalein excretion is used as an index of hepatic health, the evidence as to the effect of age is conflicting (Kampmann *et al.*, 1975).

Drugs can broadly be divided into two groups: water-soluble (polar) and lipid-soluble (non-polar). The fate of these two groups is very different. Water-soluble compounds are excreted unchanged via the kidneys. Renal function is thus all-important. Most drugs, however, are lipid-soluble: they are filtered by the glomerulus but are almost totally reabsorbed in the distal nephron. In theory, therefore, they could circulate indefinitely. In practice they are metabolized to more water-soluble compounds which are then excreted by the kidneys (Remmar, 1970).

32

For a lipid-soluble drug the rate of metabolism controls the duration of action of a single dose and the steady-state concentration reached by multiple dosing. Drug metabolites are usually less active than the parent drug. However, this is not always so; for instance, cyclophosphamide only becomes active after hydroxylation. Accumulation of pharmacologically active metabolities (such as desmethyldiazepam from diazepam) may contribute to unwanted side-effects.

For an orally administered drug to reach the systemic circulation it must first pass through the portal circulation and the liver. Many drugs are largely metabolized on this first passage through the liver (hepatic first-pass metabolism). The proportion of the drug removed by one passage through the liver is called the hepatic extraction ratio. In drugs such as propranolol or lignocaine, with a high extraction ratio, only a small proportion of the absorbed dose actually reaches the systemic circulation. This explains why the equipotent intravenous dose of such a drug is so much smaller than the oral dose, e.g. propranolol 5–10 mg intravenously; 80–90 mg orally.

Many types of biochemical reaction can take place to metabolize a drug to make it more water-soluble. Basically they fall into two main groups (Drayer, 1974; Glauser, 1974).

Phase one reactions introduce polar groups to the drug structure by, for example, reduction, oxidation, or hydrolysis. Of these reactions oxidation is by far the most important. Oxidation by hepatic microsomes is the main metabolic pathway for inactivation of most psychotropics, anticonvulsants, oral anticoagulants, and oral hypoglycaemics. Microsomal oxidation seems to be under polygenic control (Whittaker and Evans, 1970). The substantial decline in hepatic oxidation with age (O'Malley *et al.*, 1971; Vestal *et al.*, 1975) is likely to be a major factor in the increased incidence of drug toxicity in the elderly (Farah *et al.*, 1977). In 1974 Irvine *et al.* showed hydroxylation also exhibited an age-related decline, using amylobarbitone as a model. However, this result must be treated cautiously as the methodology has been criticized. Acetylation, another less important pathway, appears not to be affected by age (Farah *et al.*, 1977).

Phase two reactions involve conjugation with glucuronic acid, glycine, sulphate, or similar groups to give increased water-solubility. The two phases are not mutually exclusive. Some drugs undergo phase one then phase two reactions, whilst others only undergo phase one or phase two reactions. The metabolities formed are usually more water-soluble but are not necessarily pharmacologically inert. Most are excreted in the urine but some conjugates are excreted in the bile.

The first studies of the effect of age on hepatic enzyme function were by Kato *et al.* (1964). They were carried out in animals, so extrapolation to humans must be done with caution. The studies showed a reduction in microsomal drug metabolizing activity with age. In particular, liver cytochrome P450 was reduced. This important oxidase is easily studied because it has a typical absorption maximum at 450 nm and is simply measured. Cytochrome P450-mediated oxidations are relatively unspecific for substrates, giving high potential for drug reactions, especially by metabolism induction, and show marked variation between and within species. To date there are no studies in man comparable to these animal studies. More indirect methods have used plasma half-lives or clearance of drugs extensively metabolized by the liver. These studies have shown that the elderly have a diminished ability to metabolize a number of drugs.

The model compound antipyrine has been studied in detail. It is useful because it is minimally protein-bound and extensively oxidized in the liver. Most studies have shown a prolonged half-life and reduced metabolic clearance in older subjects (O'Malley *et al.*, 1971; Liddell *et al.*, 1975; Vestal *et al.*, 1975). However, the largest study also showed that inter-subject variation was more important than age and that only 3% of the variance in metabolic clearance could be explained by age alone (Vestal *et al.*, 1975). Studies of plasma clearance have shown an age-related reduction for phenylbutazone (O'Malley *et al.*, 1971), quinine, chlormethiazole, acetanilide (Farah *et al.*, 1977), and desmethylimipramine (Nies *et al.*, 1977). However, plasma clearance is also affected by volume of distribution and protein binding, both of which change with age. Thus this evidence for reduced metabolism with age is not definitive, though it is strongly suggestive.

Just to add a little confusion, there is evidence that not all drugs show a diminished oxidation with age, and that occasionally plasma clearance actually rises with age. Hepatic clearance of diazepam, lignocaine, and warfarin appears to be unaffected with age. Phenytoin plasma clearance may rise with age (Hayes *et al.*, 1975b) but this could be a result of changes in protein binding rather than in rates of hepatic hydroxylation and conjugation.

Not all drugs are metabolized by oxidation. The evidence regarding age-related changes in other metabolic pathways is slowly accumulating. Acetylation in the liver is the method of metabolism for drugs such as hydrallazine, procainamide, dapsone, and isoniazid. It occurs via non-microsomal enzyme pathways (Evans *et al.*, 1960). The population can be divided into fast acetylators and slow acetylators. Drug side-effects are much more common in slow acetylators. Acetylation appears not to alter with age. This has been well documented for isoniazid by Farah *et al.* (1977). Nitrazepam is metabolized by reduction then actylation. Its half-life and hepatic clearance show no age-related changes (Castleden and George, 1979). Thus the well-documented increased sensitivity to this drug in the elderly must be due to other mechanisms. Alcohol is oxidized by a non-microsomal enzyme alcohol dehydrogenase. This metabolic step is not affected by age (Vestal *et al.*, 1977). So present evidence suggests that non-microsomal enzyme pathways are less affected by ageing than microsomal pathways. Little is known about conjugation, reduction, or hydrolytic pathways.

The effect of age on enzyme induction by drugs has been studied in animals by Kato and Takanaka (1968). They showed a less marked increase in cytochrome P450 after phenobarbitone induction in elderly animals. Salem *et al.* (1978) studied the effect of a course of dichloralphenazone on the plasma clearances of antipyrine and quinine. It is likely that increased plasma clearance of these drugs is a valid within-subject index of enzyme induction (Stevensen *et al.*, 1979). The study showed a less marked increase in clearance in the elderly, implying a reduced induction response. Thus present evidence points to a reduced enzyme-inducing capacity in the elderly. This is likely to reduce chronic tolerance to drugs normally inactivated by metabolism and may contribute to the higher incidence of adverse drug reactions found in the elderly.

No direct evidence is available on hepatic first-pass clearance in the elderly. Castleden *et al.* (1975) showed much higher plasma propranolol levels after oral administration of a single dose in the elderly. Feely and Stevenson (1978) have confirmed this finding during chronic oral administration. Since propranolol has a high hepatic clearance ratio, first-class elimination is the dominant factor controlling serum levels after oral administration. Chlormethiazole has a 90% hepatic first-class elimination. Its plasma clearance is also substantially reduced in the elderly, though indices of distribution are not markedly affected by age (Nation *et al.*, 1977a). These studies suggest that hepatic first-pass elimination is likely to be reduced in the elderly.

Most studies of drug metabolism in the elderly have so far concentrated on single doses. Although this is undoubtedly interesting, the effect of repeated doses is of far greater clinical importance. Only a few studies have examined the effect of age on steady-state drug concentrations. Houghton *et al.* (1975) found a positive correlation between age and plasma phenytoin concentration. A positive age correlation also occurs with imipramine, desmethylimipramine, and amitriptyline but not nortriptyline (Nies *et al.*, 1977). Propranolol shows a four-fold increase in steady-state concentration between the ages of 40 and 70 years (Feely and Stevenson, 1978). Clearly many more studies are needed in this area.

Factors other than age are known to influence the metabolism of drugs. These factors are listed in Table 2.8. So far no studies have been undertaken to establish how they interact with age-related changes in metabolism. In particular, the animal work suggesting reduced rates of drug metabolism in females needs to be copied for humans. With the female predominance among the elderly, this sex difference could be very important.

Thus there is no uniform change in the metabolism of drugs in the elderly. Sufficient is known to be sure that a bland assumption of a generalized slowing-down of drug metabolism in old age is invalid. Detailed specific knowledge of each major drug is needed—at present we have only a few isolated examples.

Table 2.8 Factors which influence drug metabolism

Factor	Result produced
Age	Elderly/neonates (reduced metabolism)
Sex	In animal work reduced rate of metabolism in females (pregnancy—may exhibit increased metabolism)
Genetic factors	E.g. slow and fast acetylators
Environment	Increased metabolism with exposure to certain industrial chemicals
	Smoking, alcohol ⟋ acute ingestion—inhibition ⟍ chronic ingestion—induction
Diet	May be influenced by high-protein diet; decreased metabolism in starvation
Disease	Hepatic disease, particularly cirrhosis, reduced elimination

EXCRETION

Renal excretion

The age-dependent changes in renal function are probably the single most important factor in the altered pharmacokinetics of the aged, since the vast majority of drugs or their metabolities are excreted via the kidney. Before considering ageing changes, it is first helpful to consider the normal pattern of excretion.

Water-soluble (polar) drugs are excreted unchanged, whereas lipid-soluble (non-polar) drugs are filtered by the glomerulus then reabsorbed as they pass down the renal tubule. Lipid-soluble drugs require metabolism to more water-soluble metabolites before renal excretion. The main method of renal drug excretion is by glomerular filtration, although a few drugs (e.g. penicillin, probenicid, salicylates) undergo active or passive proximal tubular secretion. The three factors regulating the amount of a drug filtered through the glomerulus are the plasma concentration, the degree of protein binding and the glomerular filtration rate (GFR). As the concentration of unbound drug increases the amount filtered shows a linear increase (Caffruny, 1977). As the GFR declines, the excretion rate diminishes and the half-life may be prolonged. The practical effects of reduced excretion depend on the type of drug (Fabre and Balant, 1976). In polar compounds normally excreted unchanged the risk of high serum levels and toxicity is markedly increased, especially if the drug has a low therapeutic ratio, e.g. kanamycin. However, some drugs have compensatory mechanisms of non-renal excretion at higher serum levels (e.g. ampicillin, frusemide). With lipid-soluble drugs the chief risk of toxicity comes from an accumulation of active or toxic metabolites rather than from the parent drug. Many drugs are now known to have active metabolities which will accumulate in renal impairment and cause enhanced drug action or toxicity (Drayer, 1976, 1977). This is known to occur with procainamide, pethidine, nitrofurantoin, clofibrate, allopurinol, and other drugs.

The other main process of renal excretion is by active tubular secretion. This is affected by plasma concentration but probably not by degree of protein binding (in contrast to glomerular filtration). The drug is actively transported into the renal tubular cells then into the lumen of the tubule by a complex bidirectional carrier system (Caffruny, 1977). Two similar systems exist: one for weak acids and the other for weak bases. These pathways can be saturated. They are not substrate-specific so competition between drugs for the same pathway can exist. For instance, competition between salicylate and methotrexate can occur, and the incidence of methotrexate toxicity increases with concomitant aspirin (Henderson *et al.*, 1965).

In addition to active secretion passive tubular diffusion may occur and can sometimes be important. Here the dominant factors are pH and the rate of urine flow. As would be expected, weak acids or bases are best reabsorbed when in their unionized lipid-soluble form. Making the urine alkaline will ionize weak acids such as salicylate, which will thus be less well absorbed. This can be put to practical use in the technique of increasing salicylate excretion by forced alkaline diuresis.

Age causes a decline in most aspects of renal function, summarized in Table 2.9. Glomerular filtration rate declines by 30% between the ages of 25 and 65 years. Tubular function shows a similar decline. The reserve of renal function is greatly diminished in the elderly. Thus drug accumulation and toxicity can occur relatively easily, especially if renal function is further compromised by dehydration, congestive cardiac failure, hypotension, urinary retention, or renal disease (especially diabetic nephropathy and pyelonephritis).

Table 2.9   Changes in renal function with age

Renal mass declines by 30% (25–75 years)
Decreased renal perfusion (50% decline by 20–90 years)
Glomerular filtration rate declines ($123\,\mathrm{ml} \rightarrow 65\,\mathrm{ml/m/1.73\,m^2}$) (20–90 years)
Tubular cell function declines by 40% (25–80 years)
Increased filtration fraction
Decreased creatinine excretion ($24 \rightarrow 12\,\mathrm{mg/kg/24\,h}$) (30–80 years)
Urine specific gravity declines ($1.032 \rightarrow 1.024$) (25–80 years)
Maximum urine osmolality declines ($1040 \rightarrow 750$) (20–80 years)
Diminished response to antidiuretic hormone

The effects of changes in renal physiology with age have been confirmed by pharmacological studies. Table 2.10 shows the drugs in which detailed studies of renal handling in elderly subjects have been undertaken.

The pioneer work in this field was by Leikola and Vartia in 1957. They found that serum procaine penicillin and benzyl penicillin levels were distinctly higher in older subjects when compared to their younger controls. These drugs are excreted by active tubular secretion. Hanson *et al.* (1970) postulated that the elevation in old age was due to saturation of the excretory mechanism and to reduction in its capacity. In 1960 Vartia and Leikola produced similar results for dihydrostreptomycin and tetracycline. These findings were corroborated by Bender (1974).

In 1969 Ewy *et al.* produced a major study on digoxin kinetics in the

Table 2.10 Studies of renal drug handling in the elderly

Drug	Age-related change	Reference
Benzylpenicillin	Higher serum levels	Leikola and Vartia, 1957
Benzylpenicillin	Increased half-life	Kampmann *et al.*, 1972
Procaine penicillin	Higher serum levels	Leikola and Vartia, 1957
Propicillin	Smaller V_d	Simon *et al.*, 1972
Tetracycline	Higher serum levels	Vartia and Leikola, 1960
Dihydrostreptomycin	Higher serum levels	Vartia and Leikola, 1960
Kanamycin	Increased half-life	Lumholtz *et al.*, 1974
Gentamicin	Increased half-life	Lumholtz *et al.*, 1974
Cephalothin	Increased half-life	Kampmann *et al.*, 1974
Sulphamethiazole	Increased half-life	Triggs *et al.*, 1975
	Reduced clearance	
Digoxin	Increased half-life	Ewy *et al.*, 1969
Phenobarbitone	Increased half-life	Traeger *et al.*, 1974
Practolol	Unchanged	Castleden *et al.*, 1975
Lithium	Decreased V_d	Lehmann and Merten, 1974

elderly. They demonstrated a strong correlation between the age of the patient and the half-life of digoxin. The young subjects (20–30 years) had a digoxin half-life of 51 h, but in the elderly (73–81 years) the half-life rose to 73 h. In both groups the serum creatinine was the same but endogenous creatinine clearance fell from 122 to 56 ml/min/1.73 m^2 from the young group to the old. The findings were considered to be due to the smaller body size in the elderly subjects and the age-related drop in renal function. Falch (1973) confirmed these findings. Bloom and Nelp (1966) noted that the rate of digoxin excretion in the kidneys was inversely related to the level of blood urea.

Penicillin excretion was studied by Kampmann *et al.* (1972), examining the effect of age and probenecid. The older subjects had markedly elevated penicillin half-lives. After a 7-day course of probenecid the increase in penicillin half-life was larger in the younger group. Thus the process of active tubular secretion was less active in the elderly and more easily blocked by competitive drugs. In fact, the natural half-life of penicillin in older subjects was only marginally shorter than that obtained after an effective dose of probenecid in the younger age group.

The half-life of phenobarbitone increases 50% between youth and old age (>70 years) (Traeger *et al.*, 1974). Lumholtz *et al.* (1974) showed that the half-lives of kanamycin and gentamicin increase substantially with age. For instance, the gentamicin half-life increased from 93 min

(SD = 26 min) in the young controls to 216 min (SD = 60 min) in the elderly. One major point recurring throughout these studies is that creatinine clearance can vary widely with age, with serum creatinine remaining virtually constant. So to base drug dosages only on serum creatinine is totally unsatisfactorily (Cutler and Orme, 1969; McHenry *et al.*, 1971). It can also be misleading to use half-life measurements when the volume of distribution of the drug is altered with age. This is neatly shown in the study of Castleden *et al.* (1975) on practolol. A single oral dose produced higher practolol plasma levels in the elderly. However, this was due to altered distribution: the half-life was unchanged.

From these pharmacological studies it is clear that a very strong case exists for the modification of drug dosage in elderly patients. As a working generalization it seems that endogenous creatinine clearance is a good indicator of renal function (Fabre and Balant, 1976). In clinical practice it does not seem to be important to know whether or not the main path of renal excretion is by glomerular filtration or tubular secretion since the excretion rate, regardless of route, seems to parallel the GFR.

In practice three factors govern the need to make dosage modifications in old age. They are: (1) the proportion of drug excreted unchanged by the kidney, (2) the existence of active or toxic metabolities, (3) the drug's therapeutic safety margin.

If a drug is extensively metabolized to inactive, non-toxic metabolites (e.g. warfarin, tolbutamide) then renal function decline does not require dosage changes. However, if a drug is excreted largely unchanged (e.g. lithium, the aminoglycosides) then dosages will need to be reduced to compensate for impaired renal function.

The role of the thereapeutic safety margin can be illustrated by the contrast between the penicillins and the aminoglycosides. The very large therapeutic ratio of the penicillins ensures that toxicity reactions do not occur in the elderly person receiving standard doses even when the creatinine clearance is as low as 20 ml/min. In contrast, standard aminoglycoside does in even mild renal impairment will often produce ototoxicity (Bazra and Lauermann, 1976).

Uraemia modifies drug effects in several ways, particularly by changing body homeostasis and drug metabolism (Lowenthal, 1974; Reidenberg, 1975; Fabre and Balant, 1976). Examples include alterations in coagulation mechanisms producing increased sensitivity to anticoagulants, alterations in potassium metabolism increasing the likelihood of digoxin toxicity, and acidosis altering tissue penetration by drugs. Richet *et al.* (1975) showed that the blood–brain barrier is less effective in uraemia. Also in uraemia the kidney itself is more sensitive to drug nephrotoxicity (Fabre and Balant, 1976). Many of the changes in uraemia are similar to those produced by ageing but the comparison does not seem to have been widely explored.

Active metabolities are usually excreted almost exlusively by the kidney. Thus age-related renal impairment will particularly affect their accumulation and toxicity. However, this area is virtually unexplored. The exception is a study by Nation *et al.* (1977b) showing a significant reduction in 24-h urinary excretion of the major lignocaine metabolite 4-hydroxyxylidine in elderly subjects.

Several methods have been used to calculate dosage modifications in uraemic patients (Tozer, 1974; Dettli, 1976; Fabre and Balant, 1976; Mawer, 1976). These schedules all aim to balance the reduced elimination rate with a reduced drug dose or frequency in an effort to stop the drug gradually accumulating. Perhaps the most practical method for the elderly patient is that proposed by Tozer. He suggested a dose-adjustment factor, based on renal function and the proportion of drug excreted unchanged by the kidney. Either drug dosage or frequency is then altered by the dose-adjustment factor, or a combination of the two methods used. In drugs with a long half-life dose reduction may be preferable, but with a short half-life extending the interval between doses may be more logical. However, interval extension can cause initially toxic levels followed by sub-therapeutic levels. Often a judicious combination of dose reduction and interval extension will be the best method. Kampmann and Hansen (1979) used this approach to modify gentamicin dosage in the elderly, with considerable success.

One problem inherent in these dosage modification schedules is that they are generalizations, based on averages. They ignore completely the considerable variations between individuals in drug handling and effects. These variations are highest in the elderly. Thus the measurement of blood levels is the best control method we have, where it is available. Monitoring blood levels is current practice for digoxin, gentamicin, and anticonvulsants. Hopefully its use will spread into other areas.

In this section the urine has been seen merely as a mode of excretion. However, for antibiotics in urinary tract infection it must be a body compartment in which adequate drug levels must be obtained rather than just an excretion channel. Ball *et al.* (1977) have found lowered urine levels of mecillinam failing to clear urinary tract infections in old people with normal serum creatinine. This also occurs with amoxycillin and could well be widespread.

Biliary excretion

Some drugs, and especially their glucoronide conjugates, are excreted in the bile. This is most likely to be important if they are polar compounds with a molecular weight of more than 400 (e.g. rifampicin, ampicillin). Also biliary excretion becomes more prominent as a compensatory mechanism in some drugs when renal excretion is impaired. A few drugs such as indomethacin have an enterohepatic circulation. So far there is no evidence of any change in these mechanisms with increasing age.

ORGAN SENSITIVITY

Having considered the alterations in drug handling in the elderly, there remains a rather nebulous area of 'tissue sensitivity'. There is some definite evidence to support the theory of altered responsiveness, but in the main the evidence is anecdotal.

Most clinicians agree that the elderly exhibit a greater sensitivity to drugs acting on the central nervous system. The response of elderly subjects to barbiturates provides an excellent example (Bender, 1964). It is well documented that barbiturates can be, and often are, devastating in the elderly (Gibson, 1966; Macdonald and Macdonald, 1977). They can produce side-effects which range from mild restlessness to frank psychosis. Whilst physiological considerations and altered drug handling do play a part in these reactions when the drugs are used chronically, a similar response can occur with the first dose, implying a definitive difference in cerebral sensitivity (Evans and Jarvis, 1972). However, this view has recently been challenged by Miller and Greenblatt (1976). Many elderly subjects were subsequently persuaded to change from barbiturates to the new 'safer' hypnotics. There is now mounting evidence that many of these drugs can bring just as disastrous effects in their wake—drowsiness with chlormethiazole and diazepam occurs twice as frequently in the elderly as in the young (Boston Collaborative Drug Survey Programme, 1973); incontinence, inanition, and immobility with nitrazepam has so far only been reported in the elderly (Evans and Jarvis, 1972). This effect does not seem to be related to altered kinetics in the elderly (Castleden *et al.*, 1977). Nitrazepam depresses motor function regardless of age but it depresses cognitive function more in the elderly than in the young. Several possible explanations have been postulated, including altered homeostasis and the unmasking of unwanted effects by intercurrent disease. A recent possibility has arisen from the work of Squires and Braestrup

42

(1977). This showed specific CNS receptors for benzodiazepines. Such receptors would, by analogy with the morphine receptors and the encephalins (Snyder, 1977), imply the existence of an endogenous neurotransmitter chemically similar to benzodiazepines. If production of this falls with age then an increased sensitivity to the exogenous transmitter (i.e. benzodiazepines) would be seen.

The elderly may also have an increased tissue sensitivity to alcohol. Robertson-Tchabo *et al.* (1975) showed that healthy elderly subjects, controlled for equivalent alcohol levels, showed greater impairment of reaction time, memory, and auditory attention than the young.

From studies carried out on heparin (Jick *et al.*, 1968) and warfarin (O'Malley *et al.*, 1977) it seems that the elderly are much more sensitive to the effect of anticoagulants. In part this may be due to impaired haemostasis resulting from degenerative vascular disease. Shepherd *et al.* (1978) investigated the effects of warfarin in detail and put forward various possible explanations: altered warfarin kinetics, increased receptor sensitivity, altered vitamin K kinetics (due to relative deficiency from poor dietary intake and decreased affinity for vitamin K), and decreased receptor sensitivity to vitamin K. Shepherd *et al.* (1978) found evidence that in the elderly there are higher levels of endogenous inhibitor of clotting factor activity which may also contribute to the overall sensitivity. The overall picture obtained from these studies is that the age-related sensitivity is multifactorial and complex.

The elderly also have a high degree of sensitivity to the effects of anaesthetic agents, including intravenous and inhaled anaesthetics; opiates, particularly pethidine; as well as the phenothiazines and droperidol. The myocardium seems less resistant to the depressant effect of these drugs and less able to compensate for the peripheral vasodilation which they produce. The incidence of arrhythmias and respiratory depression associated with this group of drugs rises with age.

In 1977 Schocken and Roth studied the β-adrenoreceptors in membrane fractions of lymphocytes and found that their number showed a negative correlation with age. Vestal *et al.* (1978) also showed that resistance to the chronotropic effect of isoprenaline on the heart exhibited a similar negative correlation with age. McDevitt *et al.* (1976), using propranolol infusions, showed that there is also an *in vivo* difference in receptor affinity which has an age-specific correlation. There are also considerable age-related alterations in the pharmacokinetics of these drugs (Castleden *et al.*, 1975).

This area of altered target organ responsiveness, as distinct from change due to degeneration and disease, is one which needs a great deal more study and clarification.

It is clear from Chapters 1 and 2 that considerable care must be taken in prescribing for the elderly patient. Although this aspect will be dealt with more fully in a later chapter, some of the more important aspects deserving particular attention are outlined in Table 2.11.

Table 2.11   Principles of prescribing for the elderly

---

(1) Does the condition need drug therapy?
   Many conditions in the elderly do not require drug therapy.
   Age does not, however, preclude therapy if the patient will have an improved quality of life by virtue of therapeutic intervention.
   Use the smallest number of drugs possible. (Polypharmacy increases the risk of drug toxicity.)
   Review drug therapy regularly to enable drugs which are no longer required to be discontinued.

(2) Factors governing choice of preparation
   Risk of disease versus risk of treatment.
   Formulation and palatability.

   Size of tablet/capsule
   Colour } The more distinctive the preparation the less likely there is to be confusion. Aids identification by patient.

   Avoid complex dosage schedules—especially intermittent schedules. Where possible use once-daily medication.

(3) Dosage
   Remember body size and composition alter with age, usually requiring a dose reduction.
   Smoking habit can influence rate of metabolism and hence dosage.
   Sex—elderly women can be more at risk with some preparations, e.g. corticosteroids, phenylbutazone.
   Renal impairment may require either decreased dosage or increased dosage interval.

(4) Points
   Educate patient about disease/tablets.
   Where patient is mentally frail supervision is required.
   Ensure that patient can open the containers.
   Due to uncertain effect of food on drug biotransformation drugs should be taken in the same time relationship to food each day.
   Compliance discussed later in text.

REFERENCES AND BIBLIOGRAPHY

Acocella, G. (1978) Clinical pharmacokinetics of rifampicin. *Clin. Pharmacokinetics*, **3**, 128–43.

Ball, A. P. *et al.* (1977) Delayed excretion and prolonged elimination half-life of mecillinam in the elderly. *J. Antimicrob. Chemother.*, **4**, 385.

Bazra, M. and Lauermann, M. (1976) Why monitor serum levels of gentamicin? *Clin. Pharmacokinetics*, **3**, 202.

Beermann, B. and Groschinsky-Grind, M. (1978) Gastro-intestinal absorption of hydrochlorothiazide enhanced by the concomitant intake of food. *Eur. J. Clin. Pharmacol.*, **13** (2), 125–8.

Bender, A. D. (1964) The pharmacological aspects of ageing. A survey of the effect of increasing age on drug activity in adults. *J. Am. Geriat. Soc.*, **12**, 114–34.

Bender, A. D. (1968) Effect of age on intestinal absorption: implications for drug absorption in the elderly. *J. Am. Geriat. Soc.*, **16**, 1331–9.

Bender, A. D. (1974) Pharmacodynamic principles of drug therapy in the aged. *J. Am. Geriat. Soc.*, **22**, 296.

Bender, A. D. *et al.* (1975) Plasma protein binding of drugs as a function of age in adult human subjects. *J. Pharm Sci.*, **64**, 1711–13.

Binns, T. B. (1971) The absorption of drugs from the alimentary tract, lungs and skin. *Brit. J. Hosp. Med.*, **6**, 133.

Bloom, P. M. and Nelp, W. B. (1966) Relationship of the excretion of tritiated digoxin to renal function. *Am. J. Med. Sci.*, **251**, 133–44.

Bogentoft, C. *et al.* (1978) Influence of food on the absorption of acetylsalicylic acid from enteric coated dosage forms. *Eur. J. Clin. Pharmacol.*, **14** (5), 351–5.

Borga, O., Piafsky, K. M., and Nilsen, O. G. (1977) Plasma protein binding of basic drugs. *Clin. Pharmacol. Therapeut.*, **22**, 539.

Boston Collaborative Drug Surveillance Programme (1973) Clinical depression of the central nervous system due to diazepam and chlordiazepoxide in relation to cigarette smoking and age. *New Engl. J. Med.*, **288**, 277–80.

BP policy on dissolution testing (1978) *Pharm. J.*, **220**, 481.

Brodie, B. B. (1964) Physico-chemical factors in drug absorption and distribution of drugs. In T. B. Binns (ed.) *Absorption and Distribution of Drugs*, p. 16. Livingstone, Edinburgh and London.

Caffruny, E. L. (1977) Renal tubular handling of drugs. *Am. J. Med.*, **62**, 491.

Castleden, C. M. *et al.* (1975) The effect of age on plasma levels of propranolol and practolol in man. *Brit. J. Clin. Pharmacol.*, **2**, 303–6.

Castleden, C. M. *et al.* (1977a) Increased sensitivity to nitrazepam in old age. *Brit. Med. J.*, **1**, 10–12.

Castleden, C. M., Volans, C. N., and Raymond, K. (1977) The effect of ageing on drug absorption from the gut. *Age and Ageing*, **6**, 138–43.

Castleden, C. M. and George, C. F. (1979) Increased sensitivity to the benzodiazepines. In J. Crooks and I. H. Stevenson (eds), *Drugs and the Elderly*, pp. 169–78. Macmillan, London.

Chan, K. *et al.* (1975) The effect of age on plasma pethidine concentrations. *Br. J. Clin. Pharmacol.*, **2**, 297–302.

Crounse, R. G. (1963) Effective use of griseofulvin. *Arch. Dermatol.*, **87**, 176–80.

Cusack, B. *et al.* (1980) Effects of age and smoking on theophylline pharmacokinetics. *Br. J. Clin. Pharmacol.*, **8** (4), 348–85.

Cusack, B. *et al.* (1979) Digoxin in the elderly: pharmacokinetic consequences of old age. *Clin. Pharmacol. Ther.*, **00**, 000.

Cutler, R. E. and Orme, B. M. (1969) Correlation of serum creatinine concentration and kanamycin half-life. *J. Am. Med. Assoc.*, **209**, 539–43.

Dettli, L. (1976) Drug dosage in renal disease. *Clin. Pharmacokinet.*, **1**, 126–34.

Drayer, D. E. (1974) Pathways of drug metabolism in man. *Med. Clin. N. Am.*, **58**, 927.

Drayer, D. E. (1976) Pharmacologically active metabolites. *Clin. Pharmacokinet.*, **1**, 426.

Drayer, D. E. (1977). Active drug metabolites and renal failure. *Am. J. Med.*, **62**, 486.

Evans, D. A. P., Manley, K. A., and McKusick, V. A. (1960) Genetic control of isoniazid metabolism in man. *Brit. Med. J.*, **42**, 485.

Evans, J. G. and Jarvis, E. H. (1972) Nitrazepam and the elderly. *Brit. Med. J.*, **4**, 487.

Ewy, G. A. *et al.* (1969) Digoxin metabolism in the elderly. *Circulation*, **39**, 449–53.

Fabre, J. and Balant, L. (1976) Renal failure, drug pharmacokinetics and drug action. *Clin. Pharmacokinet.*, **1**, 99.

Falch, D. (1973) The influence of kidney function, body size and age on plasma concentration and urinary excretion of digoxin. *Acta. Med. Scand.*, **194**, 251–6.

Farah, F. *et al.* (1977) Hepatic drug acetylation and oxidation: effects of ageing in man. *Brit. Med. J.*, **2**, 155–6.

Feely, J. and Stevenson, I. H. (1978) The effect of age and hyperthyroidism on plasma propranolol steady state concentration. *Brit. J. Clin. Pharmacol.*, **6**, 446.

Fremstad, D. *et al.* (1976) Increased protein binding of quinidine after surgery. *Eur. J. Clin. Pharmacol.*, **10**, 441.

Geokas, M. C. and Haverback, B. J. (1969) The ageing gastro-intestinal tract. *Am. J. Surg.*, **117**, 881–92.

Gibson, I. I. J. M. (1966) Barbiturate delirium. *Practitioner*, **197**, 345–7.

Glauser, S. C. (1974) Drug metabolism: conjugations and multiple pathways. *Med. Clin. N. Am.*, **58**, 945.

Hanson, J. M. *et al.* (1970) Renal excretion of drugs in the elderly. *Lancet*, **1**, 1170.

Hayes, M. J., Langman, M. J. S., and Short, A. H. (1975a) Changes in drug metabolism with increasing age: phenytoin clearance and protein binding. *Brit. J. Clin. Pharmacol.*, **2**, 73–9.

Hayes, M. J., Langman, M. J. S., and Short, A. H. (1975b) Phenytoin clearance and protein binding. *Brit. J. Clin. Pharmacol.*, **2**, 251–6.

Hayes, M. J. *et al.* (1975a) Changes in drug metabolism with increasing age: warfarin binding and plasma proteins. *Brit. J. Clin. Pharmacol.*, **2**, 69–72.

Hayes, M. J. *et al.* (1975b) Changes in drug metabolism with increasing age: phenytoin clearance and protein binding. *Brit. J. Clin. Pharmacol.*, **2**, 73–9.

Hayes, M. J. *et al.* (1977) Changes in the plasma clearance and protein binding of carbenoxalone with age and their possible relationship with adverse drug effects. *Gut*, **18**, 1054.

Heading, R. C. *et al.* (1973) The dependence of paracetamol absorption on the rate of gastric emptying. *Brit. J. Pharmacol.*, **47**, 415–21.

Henderson, E. S. *et al.* (1965) The metabolic fate of nitrated methotrexate. *Cancer Res.*, **25**, 1018.

Hooper, N. D. *et al.* (1974) Plasma protein binding of diphenylhydantoin: effect of sex hormones, renal and hepatic disease. *Clin. Pharmacol. Ther.*, **15**, 276–82.

46

Houghton, C. W., Richens, A., and Leighton, M. (1975) Effect of age, height, weight and sex on serum phenytoin concentration in epileptic patients. *Brit. J. Clin. Pharmacol.*, **2**, 251–6.

Hurwitz, A. (1977) Antacid therapy and drug kinetics. *Clin. Pharmacokinet.*, **2**, 269–80.

Irvine, R. E. *et al.* (1974) The effect of age on the hydroxylation of amylobarbitone sodium in man. *Brit. J. Clin. Pharmacol.*, **1**, 42–3.

Jaffe, J. M. *et al.* (1971) Effect of dietary components on gastro-intestinal absorption of acetaminophen tablets in man. *J. Pharmaceut. Sci.*, **60**, 1646–50.

Jaffe, J. M. (1975) Effect of propantheline on nitrofurantoin absorption. *J. Pharmaceut. Sci.*, **64**, 1725.

Jenne, J. W. (1965) Partial purification and properties of the isoniazid transacetylase in human liver. Its relationship to the acetylation of *p*-aminosalicylic acid. *J. Clin. Invest.*, **44**, 1992–2001.

Jick, H. *et al.* (1968) Efficacy and toxicity of heparin in relation to age and sex. *New Engl. J. Med.*, **279**, 284–6.

Johnson, B. F. *et al.* (1978) Effect of a standard breakfast on digoxin absorption in normal subjects. *Clin. Pharmacol. Ther.*, **23**, 315–19.

Jusko, W. J. and Gretch, M. (1977) Plasma and tissue protein bindings of drugs in pharmacokinetics. *Drug Metab. Rev.*, **5**, 43–140.

Kamme, C. *et al.* (1978) Evaluation of spiramycin. *Scand. J. Infect. Dis.*, **10** (2), 135–42.

Kampmann, J. *et al.* (1972) Effect of some drugs on penicillin half life in blood. *Clin. Pharmacol. Ther.*, **13**, 516–19.

Kampmann, J. *et al.* (1974) Drug elimination and renal function. *J. Clin. Pharmacol.*, **14**, 307.

Kampmann, J. P., Sinding, J., and Moller-Jorgensen, I. (1975) The effect of age on liver function. *Geriatrics*, **30**, 91–5.

Kampmann, J. P. and Hansen, J. E. M. (1979) In Crooks, J. and Stevenson, I. H. (eds), *Drugs and the Elderly*. Macmillan, London.

Kappas, A. *et al.* (1976) Influence of dietary protein and carbohydrate on antipyrine and theophylline metabolism in man. *Clin. Pharmacol. Ther.*, **20**, 643–53.

Kato, R. and Tanaka, I. (1968) Metabolism of drugs in old rats: action of NADPH-linked electron transport and drug metabolising enzyme systems in liver microsomes of old rats. *Jap. J. Pharmacol.*, **18**, 381–88.

Kato, R. *et al.* (1964) Variation in the activity of liver microsomal drug metabolising enzymes in rats of different ages. *J. Biochem. Tokyo*, **63**, 406–8.

Klotz, U. (1976) Pathophysiological and disease-induced changes in drug volume and distribution: pharmacokinetic implications. *Clin. Pharmacokinet.*, **1**, 204.

Klotz, U. and Miller-Seyditz, P. (1979) Altered elimination of desmethyldiazepam in the elderly. *Brit. J. Clin. Pharmacol.*, **7**, 119.

Klotz, U. *et al.* (1975) The effects of age and liver disease on the disposition and elimination of diazepam in adult man. *J. Clin. Invest.*, **53**, 347–59.

Klotz, U. *et al.* (1976) Comparison of the pharmacokinetics of diazepam after single and subchronic doses. *Eur. J. Clin. Pharmacol.*, **10**, 121–6.

Kramer, P. A. *et al.* (1978) Tetracycline absorption in elderly patients with achlorhydria. *Clin. Pharmacol. Ther.*, **23**, 467.

Kraus, J. W. *et al.* (1978) Lorazepam elimination in liver disease. *Clin. Pharmacol. Ther.*, 24, 411–19.

Lehmann, K. and Merten, K. (1974) Elimination of lithium dependent of age in healthy people and patients suffering from renal insufficiency. *Int. J. Clin. Pharmacol.*, *Ther. Toxicol.*, **10**, 292.

Leikola, E. and Vartia, K. O. (1957) On penicillin levels in young and geriatric subjects. *J. Gerontol.*, **12**, 48–52.

Levy, R. H. *et al.* (1975) Pharmacokinetics of carbamazepine in normal man. *Clin. Pharmacol. Ther.*, **17**, 657–68.

Lewis, G. P. *et al.* (1971) Prednisone side-effects and serum protein levels. *Lancet*, **2**, 778–80.

Liddell, D. E., Williams, F. M., and Briant, R. H. (1975) Phenazone metabolism and distribution in young and elderly adults. *Clin. Exp. Pharmacol. Physiol.*, **2**, 481–7.

Linnoila, M. *et al.* (1975) Effect of food and repeated injections on serum diazepam levels. *Acta Pharmacol. Toxicol.*, **36**, 181–6.

Lowenthal, D. T. (1974) Tissue sensitivity to drugs in disease states. *Med. Clin. N. Am.*, **58**, 1111.

Lumholtz, B. *et al.* (1974) Dose-regimen of kanamycin and gentamicin. *Acta Med. Scand.*, **190**, 521–4.

McDevitt, D. G. *et al.* (1976) Plasma binding and the affinity of propranolol for a beta receptor in man. *Clin. Pharmacol. Ther.*, **20**, 152–7.

Macdonald, J. B. and Macdonald, E. T. (1977) Nocturnal femoral fracture and continuing widespread use of barbiturate hypnotics. *Brit. Med. J.*, **2**, 483–5.

McHenry, M. C. *et al.* (1971) Gentamicin dosages and renal insufficiency. Adjustments based on endogenous creatinine clearance and serum creatinine concentration. *Ann. Intern. Med.*, **74**, 192–9.

Malmborg, A. S. (1978) Absorption of erythromycin stearate after oral administration. *Curr. Med. Res. Opinion*, **5** (suppl. 2), 15–18.

Mather, L. E. *et al.* (1975) Meperidine kinetics in man: intravenous injection in surgical patients and volunteers. *Clin. Pharmacol. Ther.*, **17**, 21–30.

Mawer, G. I. (1976) Computer assisted prescribing of drugs. *Clin. Pharmacokinet.*, **1**, 67–78.

Melander, A. and Wahlin, E. (1978) Enhancement of dicoumarol bioavailability by concomitant food intake. *Eur. J. Clin. Pharmacol.*, **14** (6), 441–4.

Melander, A. *et al.* (1976) Reduction of isoniazid activity in normal men by concomitant intake of food. *Acta Med. Scand.*, **200**, 93–7.

Melander, A. *et al.* (1977a) Enhancement of the bioavailability of propranolol and metoprolol by food. *Clin. Pharmacol. Ther.*, **22**, 108–12.

Melander, A. *et al.* (1977b) Bioavailability of oxazepam: absence of influence of food intake. *Acta Pharmacol. Toxicol.*, **40**, 584–88.

Melander, A. *et al.* (1978) Influence of food on the absorption of phenytoin in man. *Eur. J. Clin. Invest.*, **14**, 441–4.

Miller, R. R. and Greenblatt, D. J. (1976) *Drug effects in hospitalized patients; experience of the Boston Collaborative Drug Surveillance Program. 1966–75.* John Wiley & Sons Inc., New York.

Miller, A. K. *et al.* (1977) Effect of age on the pharmacokinetics of tolbutamine in man (Abst. 5). *Pharmacologist*, **19**, 128.

Mitchard, M. (1979) Drug distribution in the elderly. In J. Crooks and I. H. Stevenson (eds), *Drugs and the Elderly*. Macmillan, London.

Mitchison, D. A. (1973). Plasma concentrations of isoniazid in the treatment of tuberculosis. In Davies and Pritchard (eds), *Biological Effects of Drugs in Relation to their Plasma Concentrations*, pp. 169–82. Macmillan, London.

Nation, R. L. *et al.* (1976) The pharmacokinetics of chloromethioazole following intravenous administration in the elderly. *Eur. J. Clin. Pharmacol.*, **10**, 407–15.

Nation, R. L. *et al.* (1977a) Plasma levels of chloromethiazole and 2 metabolites after oral administration to young and aged beings. *Eur. J. Clin. Pharmacol.*, **12**, 137–46.

Nation, R. L. *et al.* (1977b) Lignocaine kinetics in cardiac patients and aged subjects. *Brit. J. Clin. Pharmacol.*, **4**, 439.

Neu, H. C. (1974) Antimicrobial activity and human pharmacology of amoxycillin. *J. Infect. Dis.*, **129** (suppl.), 123.

Neuvonen, P. J. (1976) Interactions with the absorption of tetracyclines. *Drugs*, **11**, 45–54.

Nies, A. *et al.* (1977) Relationship between age and tricyclic antidepressant levels. *Am J. Psychiat.*, **134**, 790–3.

Nilsen, O. G., Storstein, L., and Jacobsen, S. (1977) Effect of heparin and fatty acids on the binding of quinidine and warfarin in the plasma. *Biochem. Pharmacol.*, **26**, 229.

Nimmo, J. *et al.* (1973) Pharmacological modifications of gastric emptying. Effects of propantheline and metoclopramide on paracetamol absorption. *Brit. Med. J.*, **1**, 587.

Ochs, H. R. *et al.* (1978) Reduced clearance of quinidine in elderly humans. (Abst.) *Clin. Res.*, **25**, 513A.

Odutola, T. A. *et al.* (1978) Electrolyte status in duogastrone-treated duodenal ulcer patients. *Nigerian Med. J.*, **8**, 337.

O'Malley, K. *et al.* (1971) Effect of age and sex on human drug metabolism. *Brit. Med. J.*, **3**, 607–9.

O'Malley, K. *et al.* (1977) Determinants of anticoagulant control in patients receiving warfarin. *Brit. J. Clin. Pharmacol.*, **4**, 309–14.

Parsons, R. L. *et al.* (1977) Pharmacokinetics of salicylate and indomethacin in coeliac disease. *Eur. J. Clin. Pharmacol.*, **11**, 473.

Prescott, L. F. (1974) Gastro-intestinal absorption of drugs. *Med. Clin. N. Am.*, **58**, 907.

Reidenberg, M. M. (1975) Kidney disease and drug metabolism. *Med. Clin. N. Am.*, **58**, 1059–62.

Remmar, H. (1970) The role of the liver in drug metabolism. *Am. J. Med.*, **49**, 617.

Richet, G. *et al.* (1975) Drug intoxication and neurological episodes in chronic renal failure. *Brit. Med. J.*, **2**, 394.

Richey, D. P. and Bender, A. D. (1977) Pharmacokinetic consequences of ageing. *Ann. Rev. Pharmacol. Toxicol.*, **17**, 49.

Rivera-Calimlin, L. *et al.* (1978) Effect of lithium on plasma chlorpromazine levels. *Clin. Pharmacol. Ther.*, **23**, 451.

Robertson-Tchabo, E. A. *et al.* (1975) Age differences in memory performance following ethanol infusion. (Abst. 455). *Proceedings of the 10th International Congress of Gerontology* (Jerusalem, Israel), **2**, 62.

Rowland, M., Benet, L. Z., and Graham, G. G. (1973) Clearance concepts in pharmacokinetics. *J. Pharmacokin. Biopharmacol.*, **1**, 123–36.

Salem, S. A. M. *et al.* (1978) Reduced induction of drug metabolism in the elderly. *Age and Ageing*, **7**, 68–73.

Sato, T., Miwa, T., and Tauchi, H. (1970) Age changes in the human liver of different races. *Gerontologia*, **16**, 368–80.

Schocken, D. and Roth, G. (1977) Reduced beta adrenergic receptor concentrations in ageing man. *Nature*, **267**, 856–8.

Shader, R. I. *et al.* (1977) Absorption and disposition of chlordiazepoxide in young and elderly male volunteers. *J. Clin. Pharmacol.*, **17**, 709–18.

Shepherd, A. M. M. *et al.* (1978) Age as a determinant of sensitivity of warfarin. *Brit. J. Clin. Pharmacol.*, **4**, 315–20.

Shull, H. J. *et al.* (1976) Normal disposition of oxazepam in acute viral hepatitis and cirrhosis. *Ann. Intern. Med.*, **84**, 420.

Simon, C. *et al.* (1972) Zur pharmacokinetik von propicillin bei geriatrischen patienten im vergleich zu jüngeren erwachsensen. *Dt. Med. Woch.*, **97**, 1999–2003.

Sjoholm, I. *et al.* (1979) The specificity of three binding sites as studied with albumin immobilised in microparticles. *Molec. Pharmacol.*, **00**, 000.

Smith, J. W., Seidl, L. G., and Cluff, L. E. (1966) Studies on the epidemiology of adverse drug reactions. *Ann. Intern. Med.*, **65**, 629.

Snyder, S. H. (1977) Opiate receptors and internal opiates. *Sci. Am.*, **236**, 44–56.

Squires, R. F. and Braestrup, C. (1977) Benzodiazepine receptors in rat brain. *Nature*, **266**, 732–4.

Stevenson, I. H. *et al.* (1979) In J. Crooks and I. H. Stevenson (eds), *Drugs and the Elderly*. Macmillan, London.

Storstein, L. (1976) The effect of heparin on serum protein binding of digitoxin and digoxin. *Clin. Pharmacol. Ther.*, **20**, 15.

Tozer, T. N. (1974) Nomogram for the modification of dosage regimens in patients with chronic renal impairment. *J. Pharmacokin. Biopharmacol.*, **2**, 13–28.

Traeger, A. *et al.* (1974) Zur pharmakokinetik von phenobarbital bei: erwachsensen und greisen. *Dtsch. Ges Wesen.*, **29**, 1040.

Triggs, E. J. *et al.* (1975) Pharmacokinetics in the elderly. *Eur. J. Clin. Pharmacol.*, **8**, 55.

Vartia, K. O. and Leikola, E. (1960) Serum levels of antibiotics in young and old subjects following administration of dihydrostreptomycin and tetracycline. *J. Gerontol.*, **15**, 392–4.

Vestal, R. E. *et al.* (1975) Antipyrine metabolism in man: influence of age, alcohol, caffeine and smoking. *Clin. Pharmacol. Ther.*, **18**, 425–32.

Vestal, R. E. *et al.* (1977) Ageing and ethanol metabolism. *Clin. Pharmacol. Ther.*, **21**, 343–54.

Vestal, R. E. *et al.* (1978) Reduced β-adrenoreceptor sensitivity in the elderly. (Abst.) *Clin. Res.*, **26**, 488A.

Wallace, S. *et al.* (1976) Factors affecting drug binding in plasma of elderly patients. *Brit. J. Clin. Pharmacol.*, **3**, 327–30.

Welling, P. G. *et al.* (1975) Influence of diet and food on the bioavailability of theophylline. *Clin. Pharmacol. Ther.*, **17**, 475–80.

Whittaker, J. A. and Evans, D. A. P. (1970) Genetic control of phenylbutazone metabolism in man. *Brit. Med. J.*, **4**, 323.
Woodford-Williams, E. *et al.* (1964) Serum protein patterns in normal and pathological ageing. *Gerontologia*, **10**, 86.

Section Two

Chapter 3

Drugs acting on the central nervous system

DRUGS IN THE TREATMENT OF PARKINSON'S DISEASE

Estimates for the occurrence of Parkinson's disease vary greatly, ranging from 59 per 100,000 population to 187 per 100,000 (Garland, 1952; Brewis *et al.*, 1962; Gudmundsson *et al.*, 1967). The variation is probably due to slightly differing diagnostic criteria used in the surveys. At present in the United Kingdom the incidence is thought to be near 125 per 100,000 population.

Parkinson's disease is a slowly progressive condition with 60% of patients becoming disabled between 5 and 9 years from the onset of the disease and 80% of sufferers disabled by 10–14 years (Hoehn and Yahr, 1967). There is some evidence that the later the onset of the disease the more benign is the course (Pollock and Hornabrook, 1966). The disease carries an increased mortality, approximately three times that of the general population. Although adequate treatment reduces this mortality, it still remains 1.9 times that of the general population. Therapy has no effect on the structural progression of the disease process (Sweet and McDowell, 1975).

Before logical therapy can be applied to the disease it is essential to have a clear understanding of the disease process and the neurochemistry. In 1960 Ehringer and Hornykiewicz showed that there was a deficiency of dopamine in the corpus striatum and substantia nigra of subjects with Parkinson's disease. The degree of cell loss unfortunately did not correlate with the level of dopamine deficiency (Bernheimer *et al.*, 1965). In 1961 Birkmayer and his co-workers showed that marked clinical improvement in Parkinson's disease could be achieved by giving intravenous levodopa, the immediate precursor of dopamine. Further studies produced evidence of a constant deficiency in the striatal dopamine and an associated deficiency of the enzymes involved in synthesis of dopamine (tyroxine hydroxylase and dopa decarboxylase). Homovanillic acid, a metabolite of dopamine, is also deficient. The metabolic pathway for dopamine is detailed in Figure 3.1.

The original description of the symptoms of the disease has never been bettered (Parkinson, 1817). It has been found that the severity of the akinesia correlates well with the level of dopamine deficiency in the caudate nucleus. In patients with predominantly unilateral symptoms the deficiency of dopamine has been shown to be greater in the contralateral corpus striatum. Clinically drugs which block either pre- or post-synaptic dopamine activity can produce a Parkinson-like picture, whilst drugs like the dopamine agonist bromocriptine can relieve the symptoms. The finding that anticholinergic drugs had a beneficial effect on the symptoms of Parkinson's disease implied that one further element in the disease was a relative excess of cholinergic transmission. This would result in an imbalance between the excitatory cholinergic mechanism in the brain and the inhibitory dopamine mechanism. This theory has in part been confirmed by Rinne *et al.* (1973), who found an increase in the acetyl-cholinesterase: dopamine ratio in the brains of sufferers of the disease. It has been postulated that cholinergic neurones grow in to replace the lost dopaminergic neurones (Calne, 1977).

There are undoubtedly other factors still to be elucidated. Not all patients respond to L-dopa. During prolonged administration of L-dopa a decreased response occurs. This ultimately results in levodopa-induced dyskinesia and is due to chronic denervation resulting in hypersensitivity at the receptor sites.

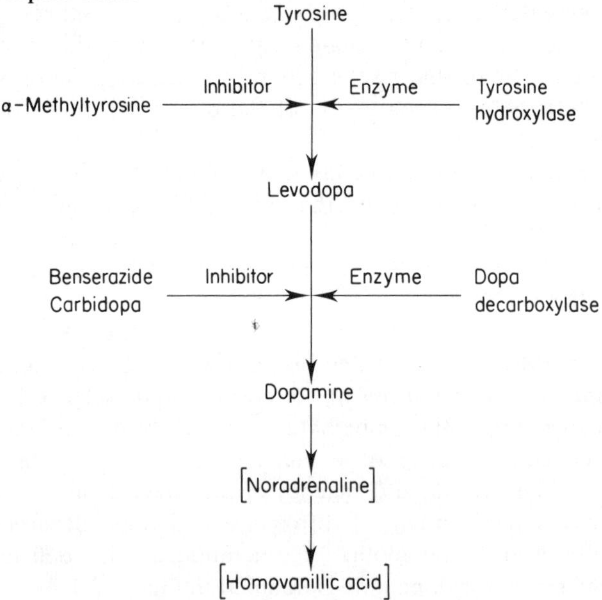

Fig. 3.1   The metabolic pathway for dopamine

Approximately 50% of patients dying of Parkinson's disease show a marked decrease in the concentration of GABA (gamma-aminobutyric acid) and in the concentration of the enzyme GAD (glutamic acid decarboxylase) required for its synthesis (Pearce, 1978). This finding seems to be an effect of the disease process rather than a cause, since therapy with a GABA analogue produces no clinical improvement. Indeed it results in an exacerbation of the clinical situation. Serotonin (5HT) is also reduced. Choline acetyltransferase activity and the binding of acetylcholine at receptor sites declines with age (Bowen and Davison, 1978).

DRUG THERAPY

There are various groups of drugs which can produce a clinical improvement in Parkinson's disease. These are listed in Table 3.1.

The solanaceous alkaloids

These were the first drugs to be tried in the disease. Hyoscine was used first in 1867 and followed by atropine and belladonna. These substances are now obsolete.

Anticholinergic drugs

These drugs entered clinical practice in the 1950s. They have largely been overtaken by levodopa as the first choice in the treatment of moderately severe idiopathic Parkinson's disease and postencephalitic Parkinsonism. They still have a role to play. Due to their ability to inhibit acetylcholine they may help to normalize the acetylcholine: dopamine balance in the brain. They have a synergistic effect with levodopa (Hughes, 1975). Anticholinergic drugs are probably still the first choice in the early stages of idiopathic Parkinson's disease and in the therapy of drug-induced Parkinsonism. Because of the synergism with levodopa, it appears to be beneficial to continue these drugs when levodopa is introduced. (The synergism outweigh the increased degradation of levopoda due to the delay in gastric emptying which anticholinergic drugs also cause.) Anticholinergic drugs also have a role where levodopa is contraindicated, e.g. in cardiac failure, arrhythmias and recent myocardial infarction. They are more effective in treating rigidity than tremor. If the patient can tolerate these drugs a 20–30% improvement in symptoms can be expected. Patients suffering from post-encephalitic Parkinsonism are able to tolerate high doses of these drugs.

Table 3.1 Drugs used in the treatment of Parkinson's disease

Drug	Starting dose	Normal daily dose	Special points
Benzhexol	1–2 mg b.d.	6–30 mg	
Benztropine	2 mg nocte	4–8 mg	Also available for i.v./i.m. use
Biperiden	1 mg b.d.	5–20 mg	Also available for i.v./i.m. use
Chlorphenoxamine	50 mg t.d.s.	200–400 mg	
Cycrimine	1.25 mg t.d.s.	5–20 mg	
Ethopropazine	10 mg q.d.s.	600–800 mg	
Methixine	2.5 mg t.d.s.	15–20 mg	
Procyclidine	2.5 mg t.d.s.	45–60 mg	
Orphenadrine	50 mg t.d.s.	200–400 mg	
Amantadine	100 mg o.d.	200 mg	Rare to exceed 300 mg
Levodopa	125 mg b.d.	1 g daily by 12 weeks	Increase by 125 mg. Used in frail elderly (Sutcliffe, 1973)
	250 mg b.d.	5 g daily	In fit elderly

Levodopa + inhibitor
  Sinemet 110 ≡ Carbidopa 10 mg and levodopa 100 mg
  Sinemet 275 ≡ Carbidopa 25 mg and levodopa 250 mg
  Madopar 125 ≡ Benserazide 25 mg and levodopa 100 mg
  Madopar 250 ≡ Benserazide 50 mg and levodopa 200 mg

Drug	Starting dose	Normal daily dose	Special points
	100–125 mg levodopa	2 g levodopa	Increase by 10 mg inhibitor
	10–12.5 mg inhibitor	200 mg inhibitor	100 mg levodopa
Piribedil	20–40 mg t.d.s.	300 mg daily	
Bromocriptine	5 mg daily	80–100 mg daily	Increase slowly. Side-effects common over 100 mg

In all instances the doses must be carefully individualized.

If mental confusion occurs in a patient taking both an anticholinergic drug and levodopa the first step is to stop the anticholinergic drug since it is more likely to be the culprit. Table 3.1 gives an indication of the dosage schedules and Table 3.2 the side-effects of the drugs.

Amantadine

This drug was introduced into the treatment of Parkinson's disease by serendipity. It was already used in the treatment of influenza when astute clinical observation indicated that it also seemed to improve Parkinson's disease (Schwab *et al.*, 1969). It is thought to work by augmenting dopaminergic function, perhaps by releasing dopamine from the remaining intact dopaminergic terminals in the basal ganglia (Stromberg *et al.*, 1970). The effectiveness of the drug tends to diminish 4–6 weeks after starting therapy. However, after stopping the drug for 2–3 weeks its effectiveness is restored. Its main role is in patients who can tolerate only a suboptimal dose of levodopa. Table 3.1 details the dosage schedule and Table 3.2 the side-effects.

Table 3.2   Side-effects of drugs used in the treatment of Parkinson's disease

Drug group	Side-effects	Points of note
Anticholinergic drugs	Drowsiness	
	Hallucinations	Estimated to occur in 20% of patients (Duvoisin, 1969)
	Confusion	
	Dry mouth	
	Blurred vision	May precipitate acute glaucoma
	Prostatism and urinary retention	Stop drug
	Constipation	
Amantadine (side-effects not common in the normal therapeutic range)	Restlessness/ giddiness	
	Insomnia/nightmares	
	Confusion	
	Hallucinations	
	Oedema	Responds to salt restriction and/or diuretics (Parkes *et al.*, 1971)
	Livedo reticularis	Usually on the thighs (Parkes *et al.*, 1971)
Levodopa	Vomiting and nausea	70–90% where levodopa alone. Do not give metoclopramide as can cause dyskinesia. Best to use cyclizine
	Confusion, hallucinations	25% of subjects. Can result in hypomania (Yahr *et al.*, 1971)
	Dyskinetic movements	26–60%. Frequently coincide with maximum improvement in mobility

Table 3.2   continued

Drug group	Side-effects	Points of note
	Increased libido	
	Hypertensive crisis if used with 4 weeks of a MAOI	
	Postural hypo-tension	20% if levodopa used without an inhibitor (Desjacques *et al.*, 1973) (helped by ephedrine 20 mg b.d.)
	Cardiac arrhyth-mias	
Piribedil	Dyskinesia	
	Mental confusion	80% (Feigenson *et al.*, 1976)
Bromocriptine	Nausea and vomiting	
	Postural hypo-tension	Teychenne *et al.*, 1978
	Mental confusion	

Levodopa

This is now the drug of choice for most patients with Parkinson's disease. It is a precursor of dopamine and can cross the blood–brain barrier. Once into the brain parenchyma it is converted to dopamine by the enzyme dopa decarboyxlase. This enzyme is also present in many other tissues (heart, gut, kidneys, etc.) resulting in a high degree of extra-cerebral metabolism of levodopa. It is for this reason that large doses of levodopa are required for clinical effectiveness. Levodopa is one of the few drugs to be absorbed by active transport. Absorption is variable and highly dependent on the rate of gastric emptying. Several methods have been tried to reduce the dose of levodopa: increasing the speed of gastric emptying, decreasing gastric acidity and modifying the patient's diet to reduce the amino acids competing for the absorptive pathway. By far the most useful and significant advance in this area was the introduction of dopa decarboxylase inhibitors (Bianchine and Shaw, 1976). Prior to the use of peripheral dopa decarboxylase inhibitors only 0.1% of the dose of levodopa reached the brain. Using an inhibitor it is possible to reduce the dose of levodopa by 80%. This reduces the incidence of nausea, and allows a more rapid therapeutic effect. The other particularly trouble-some side-effect, postural hypotension, is also reduced. Neither of the inhibitors (carbidopa or benserazide) cross the blood–brain barrier.

The rationale behind the use of levodopa is an effort to increase the level of dopamine in the basal ganglia. It is effective in the treatment of the major symptoms: bradykinesia, rigidity, tremor, posture, salivation and sebum secretion. A small number of patients show no clinical improvement (Brogden *et al.*, 1971). However, the majority of patients can expect at least a 50% improvement sustained over 2–3 years (Vignalou and Beck, 1973). Barbeau (1975) have documented evidence of 10 years' uneventful therapy. However, in the main the efficacy of therapy declines after 2 years (Shaw *et al.*, 1980) and the incidence of side-effects and the recurrence of severe depression rises markedly (Hunter *et al.*, 1973). The psychiatric side-effects of levodopa are usually the most troublesome and may indeed necessitate the withdrawal of the drug.

Unfortunately, in prolonged therapy with levodopa 50% of patients develop a new dyskinesia (Barbeau, 1973) consisting of choreo-athetoid movements, usually of the face but occasionally of the extremities, coming on 1–3 h after taking the dose. This can usually be relieved by a small reduction in the dose.

The most troublesome long-term problem is the 'on–off' effect in which periods of virtually normal function alternate with periods of akinesia and tremor (McDowell and Sweet, 1976). This problem usually appears after at least 2 years of therapy. However, there is now evidence to suggest that it occurs earlier if a dopa-decarboxylase inhibitor is being used (Marsden and Parkes, 1976). The clinical features of the 'on–off' phenomenon are early morning akinesia, freezing, end-of-dose deterioration, peak dose akinesia, and peak dose dyskinesia (Marsden and Parkes, 1976). The fluctuations are associated with swings in the serum dopa levels (Chase *et al.*, 1976). There is a particularly severe variant in which the swings occur from minute to minute. This does not seem to relate to plasma concentrations (Marsden and Parkes, 1976). It is very difficult to treat the 'on–off' phenomenon satisfactorily. As experimental work showed that it could be abolished by an intravenous infusion, a multiple small-dose regimen has been tried with limited success in clinical practice. If this is not effective the addition of bromocriptine is another possibility (Kartzinel and Calne, 1976). Dietary modification in the form of a 20–30 g daily protein diet may be helpful by reducing the competition for active transport sites.

Whilst the response to levodopa is initially very impressive and for a considerable number of patients produces a sustained improvement in

60

their clinical condition, a degree of caution must be exercised in its use. Dementia develops in approximately one-third of sufferers from Parkinson's disease by about 6 years from the onset of the illness. For many years this was thought merely to reflect the increased survival associated with treatment. However, evidence is slowly gathering to suggest that cortical atrophy and dementia may be precipitated by dopaminergic or anticholinergic drugs. It is therefore judicious to delay the start of drug therapy until the patient is beginning to find difficulty in managing his or her daily routine. The dosage should be kept at the lowest effective dose.

This cautionary note is not intended to deter people from using a successful therapy, merely to suggest that for the patient's sake great care should be taken in its application (Editorial, 1981).

The dosage schedules are detailed in Table 3.1 and the side-effects in Table 3.2.

Piribedil

This drug acts by stimulating dopaminergic receptors. It is not particularly powerful but may be a useful adjunct to levodopa (Feigenson *et al.*, 1976).

Bromocriptine

That bromocriptine can be effective in the treatment of Parkinson's disease is now well established. However its precise mode of action is still unclear. At present it is not known whether its effectiveness is due to the parent compound or to an active metabolite. Its activity seems to be due in part to pre-synaptic mechanisms in the dopamine neuronal systems (Reavill *et al.*, 1981). Its ability to increase motor activity is only apparent after a prolonged lag-phase (Teychenne *et al.*, 1981). It also has a marked influence on other cerebral mono-amine pathways (Snider *et al.*, 1976).

It is as potent as L-dopa but there are several important differences between the two drugs. Bromocriptine has the advantage of a longer biological half-life (>12 h). It has a longer duration of clinical activity. The plasma and cerebral concentrations show little fluctuation on normal dosage schedules (Friis *et al.*, 1979). Bromocriptine appears to be agonist at D_2 receptors and antagonist at D_1 receptors, whereas levodopa exhibits concentration-dependent agonist activity at both D_1 and D_2 receptors (Kebabian and Calne, 1979).

It does not appear to be clinically effective in patients unresponsive to levodopa.

Bromocriptine therapy should be considered in three main clinical situations:

(1) 'End-dose'—here bromocriptine is highly effective in reducing the amount of fluctuation and decreasing the dyskinesia of this group of patients. The levodopa dose can be reduced and it may prevent the development of the 'on–off' phenomenon.
(2) 'Early phase dyskinesia'—in these patients levodopa therapy can be reduced.
(3) 'Subsenstivity to levodopa'—bromocriptine and levodopa are synergistic when given in submaximal dosage (Kartzinel and Calne, 1976).

The initial trials of bromocriptine suggested that high doses of the drug were required for a good therapeutic effect (Parkes, 1979; Calne *et al.*, 1978). These patients were also given levodopa. In 1981 Lees and Stern reported a trial of high-dose bromocriptine therapy alone. It was effective in a substantial number of patients but its effectiveness waned after 2 years or so of therapy. In these instances levodopa therapy was not effective. The incidence of side-effects, particularly nausea, vomiting, dizziness and psychiatric upset, is considerable on high-dose therapy. Recent work by Teychenne *et al.* (1981) has suggested that it may be as effective if not more so to give bromocriptine in low doses (<14 mg/day). This study found a lag-period of 15–22 weeks before there was a response but that the overall response was as good as that achieved by the higher dosage schedules. The initial dose was 1 mg per day increased by 1 mg/week. With this lower dosage side-effects were less severe. Further evaluation of this work is required.

For doses and side-effects see Tables 3.1 and 3.2 respectively.

Occasionally where there is very marked unilateral disease stereotactic thalamotomy may be considered. If the tremor is particularly troublesome propranolol may be beneficial. It is also worth while enlisting the help of the physiotherapist, as exercising and walking education can produce significant benefits. Speech therapy can also be of value. Intonational exercises are the most beneficial (Scott and Caird, 1981).

SEDATIVES AND HYPNOTICS

Drugs acting on the central nervous system, especially those with a psychotropic effect, create more havoc in the elderly than any other group. Learoyd (1972) found that 16% of 236 admissions of patients over 65 years of age were due to the side-effects of psychoactive drugs. The prescribing of these drugs to elderly patients is fraught with hazards. The need for these drugs must be clearly established and the motives behind the prescription clearly understood. Where an elderly patient is maintained at home by relatives, disturbed sleep due to nocturnal restlessness may be the straw that breaks the camel's back. In a survey of domiciliary support (Sanford, 1975) broken sleep was the factor causing most relatives to seek the patient's admission to hospital. The reverse side of the coin is the unwarranted sedation of patients in care to ensure that they 'fit in'. Hall (1975) called it 'switching them off with the lights'. Sedatives can have a disturbing effect on behaviour and so the patient enters the vicious circle of unnecessary drug therapy leading to abnormal behaviour leading to yet more drug treatment. Not only does this result in scarce resources being wasted but the toll in human misery, both for the patient and the relatives, is enormous.

Not only does the incidence of side-effects increase with age but the side-effects themselves can be qualitatively different in the elderly. Examples of this are falls due to barbiturates (Macdonald and Macdonald, 1977), nocturnal restlessness (Exton-Smith, 1967), paradoxical excitement, barbiturate delirium (Gibson, 1966). More recently described is the picture of inanition, immobility and incontinence with nitrazepam (Evans and Jarvis, 1972).

Older patients need less sleep than the young. However, many elderly patients complain bitterly of insomnia. The precise reason for the inability to sleep must be closely scrutinized. It may be due to anxiety neurosis, organic dementia, or depression, as well as physical symptoms such as pain, cough, dyspnoea, or frequency of micturition. The cause must be discovered by a careful history of the sleep disturbance pattern. In early organic dementia, sufferers tend to exhibit nocturnal restlessness and daytime drowsiness. These patients may also suffer from hallucinations and delusions. In this instance the best therapy is not a hypnotic but a tranquillizer. In 1946 Diaz-Guerro *et al.* studied depressed patients and found that they tended to have difficulty in falling asleep and that they wakened early. This form of insomnia only responds to appropriate therapy for the depression.

Once the decision to use a hypnotic has been made the next problem lies in choosing a hypnotic drug appropriate to the aged subject. Hypnotic drugs all produce a non-selective depressant effect on the central nervous system. In small doses they are sedative and in large doses they produce sleep. Unfortunately, detailed pharmacokinetic and pharmacodynamic studies in the elderly are available in very few instances. The main group studied has been the benzodiazepines. These studies have shown that even with a particular drug family the age-dependent changes are not uniform. It is not proposed to give a list of drugs and doses for each. For this information a text such as Goodman and Gilman (1980) is recommended. It is, however, the intention of this work to give details of what age-dependent changes are known and to indicate particular problems and pitfalls for those prescribing for the elderly

SLEEP PATTERNS WITH AGE

Nearly all studies agree that with age the normal sleep patterns change. These changes are detailed in Table 3.3. It would thus appear that an older person is likely to have more trouble in falling asleep, will sleep lighter, and waken more often in the night.

Table 3.3   Alterations in sleep patterns with age

(1) Increased wakefulness
      Longer to fall asleep
      Increased number of wakenings

(2) Time spent in deep sleep is less
(3) Amplitude of the EEG delta waves of deep sleep is less
(4) REM sleep seems marginally reduced

BARBITURATES

These drugs have NO place in the treatment of insomnia in the elderly. Their only possible use is in the treatment of epilepsy and even here other possibilities should be considered. The problems caused by their use are legion (see Table 3.4). The first account of barbiturate dependence appeared in 1904 (Clarke) and the first reports of withdrawal symptoms occurred in the 1950s (Isbell, 1950; Wulff, 1959). In an excellent study by Wells (1973) it was shown that it was possible to wean patients satisfactorily from these drugs. This experience was borne out by Macdonald and Macdonald (1977) who found that it was possible to wean patients from barbiturates and in many instances discovered that by establishing a regular night-time routine, night sedation could be avoided entirely. Stopping barbiturates also substantially improved mental status. On barbiturates 39% of these patients were deemed unable to live alone, declining to only 1% after weaning off barbiturate therapy.

Table 3.4   Side-effects of barbiturates

 (1) Mental upset → frank psychosis
 (2) Postural instability
 (3) Dependence with physical withdrawal symptoms
 (4) Respiratory depression
 (5) Allergic reactions—particularly skin rashes
 (6) May precipitate attacks of porphyria
 (7) Cause folate deficiency
 (8) Arthralgia
 (9) Oral ulceration
(10) Predispose to hypothermia

BENZODIAZEPINES

The Boston Collaborative Drug Surveillance Programme (1973) found that central nervous system side-effects with benzodiazepines increased markedly with age. Drowsiness and sedation occurred twice as often in the over-70s than in the under-40s. The low serum albumin which occurs in the aged is thought to contribute in part to this (Greenblatt and Shader, 1974). Of drugs supplied on prescription and producing psychotropic problems, 50% were benzodiazepines. These age-related effects can be postulated to be due to altered drug disposition in the body, altered pharmacodynamics or receptor function.

Declining efficiency in drug elimination with age has been described by Triggs and Nation (1975). It has also been illustrated that the effect of a hypnotic drug depends on its plasma concentration. One reason for the increased sensitivity with age could be normal doses producing higher concentrations. In 1975 Klotz *et al.* showed that this was not the case for diazepam. Thus altered pharmacokinetics are not the entire explanation.

There may be impaired homeostatic mechanisms in the elderly which are unmasked by the administration of the drug. Intercurrent disease may unmask a normally trivial pharmacological action of the drug (e.g. β-blockers and bronchoconstriction). Recent research has produced a third interesting possibility. In 1977 Squires and Braestrup described specific benzodiazepine receptors in the CNS. This is probably analogous to the discovery of CNS morphine receptors and endorphins and encephalins (Snyder, 1977). The benzodiazepine receptor sites are distributed unevenly throughout the CNS. The presence of these sites implies the presence of an endogenous neurotransmitter similar to the benzodiazepines. If the production of this endogenous neurotransmitter declines with age then the subject would become more sensitive to an exogenous neurotransmitter, i.e. a benzodiazepine. It has been shown that the pharmacological effectiveness of the individual drugs as an anxiolytic agent correlates well with its displacement potency.

The individual members of the benzodiazepine group exhibit different age-related effects. These changes relate to alterations in their volume of distribution, changes in half-life, presence and accumulation of pharmacologically active metabolites (see Table 3.5).

Table 3.5   Benzodiazepine handling with age

	Elimination half-life in elderly	Active meta-bolites	Changes with age	Site of metabolism
Diazepam	65 h +	+	Marked increase in plasma half-life Metabolites detected later Altered initial distribution space Altered steady-state distribution volume	Liver; meta-bolites can accumulate
Chlordiaze-poxide	10–45 h	+	Increased plasma half-life Metabolite peak lower Significant reduction in total plasma clearance Increased steady-state volume of distribution	Liver; meta-bolites can accumulate
Lorazepam	16–24 h	−	No change in half-life No change in distribution Variability of plasma binding of lorazepam	Liver
Oxazepam	6–25 h	−	No change in half-life	Liver
Flurazepam	Approx. 3 h	+ +	Unknown	Liver; meta-bolites accumulate

Table 3.5   continued

	Elimination half-life in elderly	Active meta-bolites	Changes with age	Site of metabolism
Nitrazepam	15–70 h	?	No change in metabolism, but brain becomes more sensitive to lower levels Special inanition syndrome only in elderly	Liver
Medazepam	~14 h	+	Slight increase in plasma half-life	Liver; metabolites can accumulate
Triazolam	Unknown (4.5 h in young)	+	Unknown	Liver; active metabolites have short half-lives in young

Diazepam

This was first synthesized by Sternback and Reeder, and marketed in 1963. By 1972 there were 77 million prescriptions per annum for diazepam in the United States (cost $200m). The number and cost of prescriptions is still rising. In the USA 30% of all hospital inpatients receive diazepam (Greenblatt and Shader, 1974). In the UK similar trends are seen.

Diazepam is biotransformed into active metabolites. The first step is dealkylation to desmethyldiazepam, followed by hydroxylation to oxazepam. Glucuronide conjungation is the final step prior to urinary excretion. The half-life of diazepam shows an age-dependent decline from 20 h at age 20 years to 90 h at age 80 years. The metabolities take longer to appear. Their peak concentration is lower and the rate of decline slower. The total plasma and blood clearance are not significantly age-related. These findings imply an altered volume of distribution rather than an age-related change in metabolism. The initial distribution space and the distribution volume at steady state show a linear age-linked decline (Klotz et al., 1975). No change was noted for diazepam protein binding or distribution between plasma and red blood cells.

The other factor affecting central nervous system depression with diazepam (and chlordiazepoxide) is smoking habit. The Boston Collaborative Drug Surveillance Programme (1973) found that those with high tobacco consumption were less likely to have central nervous system side-effects. No obvious change in metabolism was noted between smokers and non-smokers; so other as yet unexplained factors must be in operation. Another social habit affecting diazepam metabolism is drinking: concomitant alcohol administration slows down diazepam absorption.

The dose of diazepam required for cardioversion is critically governed by the age of the subject. Reidenberg (1978) found that lower doses and lower plasma levels were required in the elderly to achieve central nervous system depression.

Chlordiazepoxide

This drug has chemical and pharmacological properties closely related to diazepam. It also undergoes similar biotransformation producing pharmacologically active metabolites. The Boston Drug Programme found little difference between chlordiazepoxide and diazepam with regard to the incidence of age-related side-effects. With advancing years the post-distributive half-life of chlordiazepoxide declines from around 6 h at 20 years to 36 h at 80 years. The time for metabolities to appear in the blood is not delayed but the peak levels are lower. Prolongation of the half-life is associated with a significant reduction in the plasma clearance. This declines from 30 ml/min at age 20 years to 8 ml/min at age 80 years (Wilkinson, 1979). There is no apparent alteration in binding or distribution between the erythrocytes and plasma. There is also an age-dependent decline in the volume of distribution of the drug. This decline is, however, only exhibited by the steady-state volume and not by the initial distribution space which remains unchanged. These factors all indicate that the half-life prolongation is in this instance both due to altered distribution and a significant reduction in the capacity of the aged liver to metabolize the drug. This serves to produce a much more marked age change than with diazepam.

Lorazepam

Wilkinson (1979) studied lorazepam to elicit any possible pharmacokinetic changes with age. The main route of metabolism for this drug is glucuronide conjugation. No age-related changes in post-distributive half-life, total plasma clearance, drug distribution or metabolite levels were found. A trend towards decreased protein binding with age was found, but the number of subjects in the group was small so this observation must be treated with caution.

Nitrazepam

This benzodiazepine is metabolized by a nitro-reduction to an amine metabolite. This is followed by acetylation. The acetylation is genetically controlled, with a fast and slow phenotype (Karim and Price-Evans, 1976). The drug is normally 90% protein-bound. The elderly seem curiously sensitive to nitrazepam despite the fact that age seems to have no effect on the disposition of nitrazepam (Castleden *et al.*, 1977). This leads to the conclusion that the elderly brain is in some way hypersensitive to nitrazepam. This may be where the benzodiazepine receptors play a role. Nitrazepam depresses motor function regardless of age, but cognitive function more in the elderly than in the young. Bond and Lader (1972) showed that there were two distinct facets to psychomotor testing. The speed with which these tests can be completed depends on motor function, whereas accuracy depends on cognitive function. The elderly do not seem to develop tolerance to nitrazepam (Adam *et al.*, 1976) although they initially have poor sleep after stopping the drug. This is in contradistinction to choral and glutethimide which become less effective with age (Adam *et al.*, 1976). Evans and Jarvis (1972) described a syndrome of disability which occurs only in elderly patients. It is characterized by immobility, incontinence, and confusion. It may appear in patients taking nitrazepam previously without ill effect. One 5 mg dose can, however, be enough to cause it, although 2.5 mg nocte does not appear to produce this picture. Fortunately, the condition reverses rapidly and completely when the drug is removed.

Flurazepam

The biotransformation of this drug is extremely rapid, the parent drug being virtually undetectable in the blood. The principal metabolities are metabolically more potent than the parent drug and have long half-lives (20–24 h). They accumulate and are probably the main contributors to the drug's toxicity. This toxicity rises with age and with increasing dosage. The incidence of adverse reactions is 1.9% in the under-60s rising to over 7% by the age of 70 years (Greenblatt *et al.*, 1977).

Oxazepam

The absorption of oxazepam is relatively slow, which may limit its use as a hypnotic. Its biotransformation is relatively simple, involving a glucuronidation to an inactive metabolite (Greenblatt *et al.*, 1975). Age does not alter the elimination half-life or the plasma clearance of oxazepam. Declining renal function does not impair the renal excretion of oxazepam but the excretion of the inactive metabolites is related to the creatinine clearance, raising the elimination half-life. Goldstein *et al.* (1978) found that the elderly tolerated oxazepam well and that there was significantly less 'hangover' with this drug than with flurazepam or chloral hydrate.

Temazepam

Temazepam appears to be absorbed faster by the old but to be eliminated rather more slowly, with an elimination half-life of about 14 h (Briggs *et al.*, 1980). This longish half-life suggests that accumulation is likely with repeated daily doses. In acute use, temazepam appears to give few 'hangover' problems the next day but long-term studies are needed to assess the effect of accumulation.

Triazolam

Triazolam has a shortish half-life of about 4.5 h in young subjects (Metzler *et al.*, 1977) but its half-life in old people is not known. One of its principal metabolites (the 1-OH methyl derivative) has considerable hypnotic activity but it probably also has a shortish half-life, at least in the young. Several studies have shown that triazolam is an effective hypnotic in old people with fewer 'hangover' effects than more long-acting benzodiazepines. These studies used doses of 0.25 mg and 0.5 mg but one recent paper has shown that 0.125 mg may well be effective in old people (Lipani, 1978).

The use of triazolam was recently suspended in the Netherlands following allegations of bizarre reactions to the drug in one centre. No similar reactions have been reported from elsewhere and other national drug authorities are satisfied with the drug's safety.

CHOICE OF HYPNOTIC

Choosing a good hypnotic for an elderly person is not easy. There is not infrequently a disparity between the properties one would expect from a drug's pharmacokinetic profile and the properties found in clinical practice. For instance, lorazepam is absorbed relatively slowly but a good clinical trial in the elderly has shown that it induces sleep relatively rapidly after ingestion. Also one would predict that flurazepam, with its ultra-rapid metabolism and active long-lived accumulating metabolites, would be a poor hypnotic with serious 'hangover' problems in old people. But in practice it has performed well. Thus in choosing a hypnotic clinical data need to take precedence over pharmacokinetic considerations.

Of the benzodiazepines, the best are probably flurazepam, oxazepam, and small doses of nitrazepam. Chlormethiazole has been extensively studied in the elderly. It is a good sleep-inducer and has very few 'hangover' effects. It should thus be a leading contender. Of the chloral derivatives, triclofos is probably the most suitable. It remains a good second-line drug, with physical dependence reported after long-term use as a drawback.

OTHER SEDATIVES/HYPNOTICS

Chlormethiazole

Several studies have been done to investigate the handling of this drug in the elderly. The main alterations with age appear to be:

(1) increased half-life (Nation *et al.*, 1976);
(2) decreased plasma clearance;
(3) decreased cell binding;
(4) increased volume of distribution (Nation *et al.*, 1976);
(5) decreased protein binding.

Hepatic metabolism is the main route of removal for the drug (Moore *et al.*, 1975) so alterations in hepatic blood flow with age could have important clinical repercussions. The Boston Collaborative Drug Surveillance Programme (1973) noted that drowsiness became more common with this preparation in older subjects. However, in two studies carried out specifically in old people (Pathy, 1977; Exton-Smith and Witts, 1979) this was not found to be a problem. The drug produced good clinical relief of insomnia with very few side-effects and virtually no 'hangover' effect. Few elderly patients seem to suffer from the intense nasal irritation which is a feature of this drug when used in younger subjects. This drug has also the advantage of being prepared as a syrup. Normal dose in the elderly is 250–500 mg. There is some evidence to suggest that dependence may result with prolonged usage (Exton-Smith and Maclean, 1979).

Chloral hydrate and dichloralphenazone

These have long been thought to be relatively safe drugs to use in the elderly. It is the experience of the authors that both these drugs can produce considerable problems with 'hangover' and particularly with postural hypotension if sleep is disturbed during the night, e.g. rising to go to the toilet (Macdonald, in press).

Table 3.6   Doses of suggested hypnotics in the elderly

Chlormethiazole	1–2 capsules (192–384 mg chlormethiazole base) (also available as a syrup: 250 mg/5 ml)
Nitrazepam	2.5–5 mg
Flurazepam	5–15 mg
Oxazepam	10–15 mg
Triclofos	1.5 g

Note: Aim to use short courses only.

ANTIDEPRESSANTS

Depression is common. It can be a difficult clinical diagnosis to establish as there is often an overlay of anxiety. The incidence of depression rises with age, as does the frequency of episodes in recurrent depressive illness. There is no one definite group of signs and symptoms. Physical illness such as early senile dementia and the effects of other drugs need to be excluded. It is then necessary to discover the nature of the depression and to bear in mind that not all depressions are helped by drugs. Depression can be reactive or endogenous. The reactive depressions may show slow spontaneous resolution (Hollister *et al.*, 1967). Endogenous depression appears to be due to a genetic biochemical abnormality and as such should be amenable to drug therapy (Weil-Malherbe and Szara, 1971). It tends to run a relapsing course. Less common in the elderly is the depression associated with manic-depressive illness. The next decision is whether to treat the patient as an inpatient or outpatient, or under the care of a general physician or psychiatrist. A detailed history is also required (Ashcroft, 1975).

Some 40 antidepressant preparations are at present available in the UK. The drugs and dosages must be carefully selected and not all depressions require antidepressants. The classical retarded or endogenous depression is the one most likely to respond to the tricyclic antidepressants. However, many patients fail to respond. There is a high incidence of adverse reactions with toxic confusional states, cardiotoxicity, and postural hypotension being among the more serious. In agitated depression an antipsychotic drug many be the drug of choice. ECT can still have a useful place in severe depression when drugs have failed.

TRICYCLIC ANTIDEPRESSANTS

The tricyclic antidepressants are the most important and most widely used of the antidepressant drugs. The group has three main pharmacological actions which the individual drugs possess to varying degrees. These effects are:

(1) Sedative: the tertiary amines (e.g. amitriptyline) have the greatest sedative effect and protryptiline has the least.
(2) Peripheral and central anticholinergic effect: amitriptyline is the strongest anticholinergic and desipramine the least.
(3) Ability to block the amine pump (the active transport mechanism which recaptures released neurotransmitters into the presynaptic nerve endings) (Axelrod, 1971). This action would appear to be the most important in respect of the antidepressant activity of the tricyclics (Baldaressini, 1975).

The main neurotransmitters in the limbic system, which deals with emotion, are serotonin and noradrenaline. They have been found to be considerably lowered in the depressed (Williamson, 1978). They also show an age-related decline and this in part may explain the increased incidence of depression in the elderly. Reserpine-induced depression appears to be due to the depletion of amine neurotransmitters, both serotonin and noradrenaline. This has produced the amine theory of depression in which both serotonin and noradrenaline play a part (Maas, 1975). This has been further supported by the fact that, although the three major groups of antidepressants (tricyclics, MAOIs, and sympathomimetics) act by different methods, they all increase neurotransmitter amines. Not all the tricyclic drugs have the same effect on the amine pump. The tertiary amines such as amitriptyline and imipramine have a more marked inhibiting effect on the serotonin pump whilst the secondary amines such as nortriptyline and desipramine have a greater effect on the noradrenaline pump (Carlsson *et al.*, 1969; Sjoqvist, 1975). However, not all the tricyclics exhibit this action. Pinder *et al.* (1977) found that the newer drug doxepin has a relatively weak action on the noradrenaline pump. Mianserin has presynaptic α-adrenoreceptor blocking activity with antihistamine activity but no central anti-cholinergic effect (Brogden *et al.*, 1978). Nomifensine inhibits the dopamine pump and the noradrenaline pump. It may therefore be that the overall balance is more important than the status of any single neuro-transmitter.

Current research suggests it might be possible to decide which particular amines are most involved and thus choose the most appropriate anti-depressant. This involves estimating the urinary excretion of 3-methoxy-4-hydroxyphenylglycol (MHPG), a metabolite of noradrenaline which arises largely from central adrenergic activity. Where MHPG is found to be low a drug to block the noradrenaline pump may be best, and where it is high or normal serotoninergic transmission is thought to be at fault. Unfortunately these techniques are not yet clinically available and they need further evaluation (Schildkraut, 1974; Beckman and Goodwin, 1975).

At present the first choice of tricyclic antidepressant would probably be a tertiary amine such as amitriptyline or imipramine, as there is evidence to suggest that depression due to deficiency in serotoninergic transmission is the more common. Amitriptyline is the most specific inhibitor of the amine pump for serotonin. The metabolite of imipramine, desipramine, more effectively blocks the pump mechanism for noradrenaline. Imipramine may be substituted where amitriptyline is causing sedation or excessive anticholinergic effects. Some of the newer drugs such as doxepin, mianserin, and nomifensine seem to produce less cardiotoxicity. They are also claimed to have less marked anticholinergic effects.

Following repeated doses of tricyclics plasma drug concentration rises until a steady-state plateau is reached (Hammer and Sjøqvist, 1967). Asberg (1974b) noted that for the same dose of nortriptyline there was tremendous inter-individual variation in the steady-state levels reached. Similar findings have been noted for imipramine (Moody and Tait, 1967); desipramine (Sjøqvist *et al.*, 1969); amitriptyline (Braithwaite *et al.*, 1972); protriptyline (White, 1976); and clomipramine (Mellstrom and Tybring, 1977). These findings are clinically relevant because of the close relationship between the plasma levels and the therapeutic and toxic effects (Asberg *et al.*, 1971; Montgomery *et al.*, 1978; Asberg, 1974b). Sjøqvist *et al.* (1969) suggested that the steady-state level is controlled by the rate of hepatic metabolism. This appears to be genetically determined although it can be modified by environmental factors, particularly previous drug exposure (Alexanderson *et al.*, 1969). In 1977 Nies *et al.* reported a positive correlation between age and steady-state plasma levels of antidepressants. There is also an increased tendency with age towards variability in the levels reached (Braithwaite *et al.*, 1978). In both older volunteers (Alexanderson, 1973) and patients (Braithwaite *et al.*, 1978) there is also an increase in the half-lives.

Recent work (Asberg *et al.*, 1971; Kragh-Sørensen *et al.*, 1973, 1976; Ziegler *et al.*, 1976; and Montgomery *et al.*, 1978) has shown that antidepressants have a circumscribed therapeutic range, e.g. 50–150 ng/ml for nortriptyline. If the levels achieved fall outside this range then the clinical results are poor. Indeed it has been shown that high levels of nortriptyline may negate the antidepressant effect of the drug, and thus allow the symptoms to persist (Montgomery *et al.*, 1978). High plasma levels are also associated with increased toxicity (Asberg, 1974b). Particularly important are the cardiotoxic effects. It is clear that the introduction of routine measurement of plasma antidepressant levels could produce substantial clinical dividends.

Table 3.7 summarizes the dosage schedules, Table 3.8 problems in the elderly, and Table 3.9 the side-effects of tricyclic antidepressants.

Table 3.7   Antidepressants

Drug	Half-life (hours)	Active metabolites	Starting daily dose in elderly (mg)	Normal adult range (mg)	Note
Amitriptyline	32–40	+ (may accumulate)	50	75–200	Half-life raised in elderly
Imipramine	6–20	+	30	100–200	
Nortriptyline	15–90	−	20	75–150	
Desipramine	12–54	−	25	100–200	
Clomipramine	17–28	−	10	30–150	
Doxepin	8–25	−	25	75–150	
Maprotiline	27–58	+	25 (nocte)	25–300	
Mianserin	8–19	−	30 (nocte)	90–200	
Nomifensine	3–5	+	25 (b.d.)	50–200	

All the above have hepatic metabolism.

The first symptom to show improvement is usually the sleep pattern. Full remission can be slow and the observers are often more aware of the

Table 3.8 Particular points to consider when using antidepressants in the elderly

---

(1) Regular ECG monitoring
(2) Be vigilant about side-effects
(3) Choice of drug is still largely empirical
(4) Dosage schedule must be tailored to each patient; the elderly nearly always require reduced dosage—usually half to one-third the accepted adult range
(5) Monitor duration of therapy carefully and where possible measure plasma levels
(6) May need to consider other therapy

Table 3.9 Side-effects of antidepressants

---

(1) Dry mouth
(2) Blurred vision
(3) Sweating
(4) Constipation
(5) Delayed ejaculation
(6) Urinary retention ⎱ Medical emergencies
(7) Paralytic ileus ⎰ May require bethanecol
(8) Toxic delirium
(9) Postural hypotension
(10) Tremor (if very troublesome may be helped by a small dose of propranolol)
(11) Weight gain—common
(12) Cholestatic jaundice ⎱ Rare
     Agranulocytosis ⎰
(14) Cardiac abnormalities
     Non-specific 'T'-wave changes
     Cardiac arrhythmias
(15) Hyperpyrexia in overdosage
(16) Unsteady gait—can be very important in the elderly

Notes:
  (i) Mianserin and nomifensine seem less likely to be caradiotoxic or produce postural hypotension.
 (ii) All cases of tricyclic antidepressant overdose should be admitted to hospital and preferably an intensive care unit.
(iii) Increased risk of anticholinergic effects if administered with other anticholinergic drugs: e.g. antihistamines; drugs used in Parkinson's disease; drugs used in therapy of peptic ulcer.

early improvements than the patient (Oswald *et al.*, 1972). If this is the first attack and remission is rapid it may be possible to taper off the drug, monitoring carefully for relapse. However, if the depression is severe and is the latest in a series of bouts slowly becoming more severe then maintenance therapy may well be indicated.

MONOAMINE OXIDASE INHIBITORS (MAOIs)

These drugs appear to be beneficial in the category of 'atypical' depression described by Johnson (1975) as anxiety with phobic features and hypochondriasis. This group of drugs functions as an antagonist of monoamine oxidase, which causes intracellular degradation of noradrenaline, adrenaline, dopamine, and 5HT. They take 2–4 weeks to become effective and persist for 2–3 weeks after stopping therapy. There are two main groups:

(1) the hydrazines: iproniazid, isocarboxazid, phenelzine, and niamid;
(2) non-hydrazines: pargyline, tranylcypromine.

They require large initial doses and small daily doses as it is necessary to produce total inhibition before improvement occurs (Robinson *et al.*, 1978). Phenelzine has genetically determined slow and fast acetylators. This seems to influence the clinical outcome with slow acetylators having a better therapeutic response. Table 3.10 gives prescribing information and Table 3.11 potential side-effects.

Table 3.10   Monoamine oxidase inhibitors (MAOIs)

Drug	
Iproniazid	100–150 mg daily in one dose, reducing to 25–50 mg daily maintenance
Isocarboxazid	30 mg daily loading doses, 10–20 mg maintenance
Phenelzine	15 mg three or four times daily
Niamid Pargyline	Not used in the elderly
Tranylcypromine	10 mg b.d. (not after 4 p.m.) Maintenance 10 mg daily

Notes:
 (i) Improvement may not show for 3–4 weeks.
(ii) Must *not* give tricyclic antidepressants for at least 14 days after stopping MAOI.

Table 3.11 Side-effects of monoamine oxidase
inhibitor antidepressants

(1) Postural hypotension
(2) Bradycardia
(3) Bowel upsets
(4) Hyper-reflexia, hyperpyrexia, convulsions
(5) Tremor, sweating
(6) Agitation → hypomania
(7) Constipation
(8) Giddiness, visual upsets, dry mouth
(9) Vasculitis
(10) Peripheral neuritis } Iproniazid especially

Note: The dietary exclusions must always be stressed, especially cheese, coffee, beef, or yeast extracts (e.g. Bovril, Oxo, or Marmite), chocolate, and cream.

Lithium

Lithium is subject to rapid oral absorption and clinical levels should be estimated 12 h after the last oral dose. It is not protein-bound and is distributed in the total body water. Its slow entry into cells accounts for its delayed clinical onset. No metabolism of lithium occurs as virtually all the ion is excreted unchanged via the kidney. Modest amounts of lithium are excreted in the sweat in hot weather. Renal clearance of lithium correlates well with creatinine clearance (Mason *et al.*, 1978). Toxic concentrations can occur in the distal and collecting tubules. If sodium is depleted lithium clearance declines. It can be reduced by almost 25% in the presence of thiazide diuretics. If a thiazide diuretic has to be used at the same time a decrease in the lithium dose is imperative.

Hewick *et al.* (1977) found the steady-state plasma concentration to be higher in the elderly. This is due to a decreased volume of distribution and to a diminished rate of renal clearance in the elderly (Lehmann and Merten, 1974). Table 3.12 gives doses and clinical applications in the elderly, and Table 3.13 side-effects.

Table 3.12 Lithium

Normal dose	Range	Excretion	Side-effects
0.25 g Start	600 mg–3.6 g	Kidney	See Table 3.13
Increase dose slowly till within therapeutic range			

78

Special points to Table 3.12:
(a) Plasma level:
    0.8–1.0 mmol/l, 12 h after previous dose; toxicity at 1.5 mmol/l and above.
(b) Plasma levels influenced by:
    renal function—this is important in the old;
    upsets in body sodium;
    alterations in gastric emptying.
(c) Must measure blood levels at least every 6 weeks and thyroid function every 3 months.
(d) Baseline renal function estimation necessary.

Table 3.13   Side-effects of lithium

(1) Tremor	Common; may require propranolol
(2) Ataxia, dysphasia, dysarthria, confusion, unusual movements	Can occur with therapeutic doses
	Reduce dose and gives four times daily instead of three times
(3) Nausea, vomiting, abdominal pain	Give four times daily
(4) Hypothyroidism, goitre	Reversible with thyroxine; late onset
(5) Nephropathy	Occurs with prolonged therapy
(6) Renal tubular disease	Occurs early in therapy; may become polyuric
(7) Occasionally nephrogenic diabetes insipidus	
(8) Oedema and weight gain	
(9) Acne and folliculitis	Usually resolves
(10) Occasional cardiac abnormalities	T-wave changes; arrhythmias

CEREBRAL ACTIVATING DRUGS

Dementia has a devastating effect both on the sufferers and those members of the patient's family who have to watch the disintegration of the personality of someone dear and close to them. For every one patient suffering from dementia in an institution or hospital there are estimated to be five more sufferers in the general population (*BMJ* Editorial, 1974). The prevalence rises from 2% in the 65–75 age group to 20% in those over 80 years.

The market for effective drugs acting on the nervous system is potentially very large. At present cerebral activating drugs are amongst the most widely prescribed and financially lucrative drugs on the market (Lloyd-Evans *et al.*, 1978).

With age the cerebral blood flow and the autoregulatory mechanisms become vulnerable. The old become less able to maintain their cerebral perfusion, especially if the haematocrit rises. Cerebrovascular disease results in a fall in the cerebral blood flow. Dementia also produces a decline in the cerebral blood flow. Initially this was thought to be a cause of dementia but recent work has shown that the decreased flow is secondary to the decreased metabolic demands of cerebral tissue.

In normal old age the cerebral metabolic requirement for oxygen ($CMRO_2$) is unchanged. If the oxygen supply is reduced then there is a consequent reduction in adenosine triphosphate (ATP). The repercussions of this are very important as ATP and cyclic adenosine monophosphate (c-AMP) influence the calibre of the cerebral arterial tree (Forrester *et al.*, 1975; Flamm *et al.*, 1975). It also appears that the cyclic nucleotides are involved in the memory process (McIlwain, 1977). The reduction in $CMRO_2$ is related to the degree of dementia.

Before prescribing drugs in the hope of improving dementia it is essential that all potentially reversible causes of mental clouding and confusion should be excluded (e.g. infection, drug therapy, metabolic upsets, etc.). In younger patients some 10–20% of cases of confusion will have a reversible cause. Unfortunately, in the very elderly this is unlikely to be so, but it is still very well worth while to search for the few reversible cases. Pseudo-dementia secondary to depression must always be borne in mind.

There is considerable interest at present in the biochemistry of dementia and the anatomical changes found in the brains of demented subjects. The consensus of opinion at present seems to be that the primary defect is in the metabolism of choline with a deficit of choline acetyltransferase (Glen, 1980). This is not the sole factor and there are thought to be other contributing defects. The aim of this research is to find a specific replacement therapy similar to that of L-dopa in Parkinson's disease. Unfortunately, at present such a therapy is not available and the doctor is left with the rather nebulous vasodilator/cerebral activating drugs. These drugs can be divided into three main groups:

(1) simple cerebral vasodilators;
(2) cerebral 'activating' drugs which are believed to influence both the cerebral circulation and the cerebral metabolism;
(3) drugs influencing neuronal metabolism but having no effect on the cerebral circulation.

Group 1: simple cerebral vasodilators—isoxuprine (Duvadilan); cyclandelate (Cyclospasmol)

The value of these drugs was based on the false assumption that decreased perfusion caused dementia rather than resulted from the dementing process. Isoxuprine has not been shown to have any beneficial action at all, and indeed by reducing the cerebral perfusion may actually be harmful. Cyclandelate has, because of its direct action on smooth muscle, been postulated as beneficial in vascular dementia. This has not been shown to be the case (Goodman and Gilman, 1980).

Group 2: cerebral activators which influence the vasculature

The theory behind these drugs is that by improving the utilization of glucose and oxygen in the brain they will improve the function of the compromised brain.

Dihydroergotoxine mesylate (Hydergine) acts by α-blockade. In animal research it has been shown to influence enzymes involved in the intermediary stages of metabolism in the ganglion cells. In several clinical studies it has been shown to exert no effect despite some alteration detectable on the EEG. This drug is not without risk. It is an ergot compound and prolonged use can result in peripheral gangrene, especially if there is pre-existing peripheral vascular disease (Goodman and Gilman, 1980). It can also produce sinus bradycardia and hypotension.

Naftidrofuryl (Praxilene) has been shown to influence cerebral metabolism in several ways: an increase in adenosine triphosphate and a reduction in the concentration of lactic acid (Meynaud, 1975). It has been shown to improve memory but not so far to improve the activities of everyday living (Yesavage, 1979).

There is a third drug in this group—pentifylline. It is thought to increase the cerebral uptake of glucose. At present there is no real evidence of this drug's clinical usefulness.

Group 3: cerebral activators with no vasodilator effect

These drugs are believed to influence neuronal metabolism. So far the two main drugs in this group have not been fully evaluated.

Meclofenoxate (Lucidril) is thought to reduce the cerebral oxygen requirement (Gedye *et al.*, 1972) and pyrtinol hydrochloride to increase cerebral perfusion (Flood, 1979).

At present it is doubtful if these drugs make a worthwhile contribution to the management of patients with dementia.

Much has been written recently about the possible role of levodopa in the treatment of dementia. The evidence so far is conflicting. Lewis *et al.* (1978) found marked improvement in elderly patients treated with doses starting at 125 mg daily rising gradually over 2 weeks to 875 mg daily. They found, however, that the improvement in intellectual function did not extend into the functions of everyday living. These lines of research are of great interest but so far of limited practical importance.

It is very important that the prescribing of doubtful drugs does not lull the medical practitioner into a false sense of security, obscuring other more important facets of treatment. Where these patients are being cared for at home they place a great strain on their families. Good social support is essential: holiday relief, washing services if incontinence is a problem, etc. Support groups for families can also be a great boon. It behoves all doctors involved with this problem to deal with it with compassion and to press for adequate provision of essential support services.

STROKE

Various approaches have been used in an effort to limit the damage caused by stroke. Studies on cerebral vasodilators have been inconclusive; some agents improve cerebral blood flow in stroke but none has shown a clear clinical benefit. Corticosteroids, glycerol, and mannitol have been recommended to reduce the cerebral oedema which accompanies infarction. Glycerol and mannitol can sometimes relieve the situation temporarily in massive cerebral infarction by dehydrating normal brain tissue and reducing the risk of tentorial herniation. Corticosteroids appear to have no effect in reducing the oedema of cerebral infarction (Mulley *et al.*, 1978). Also there is no convincing evidence that drugs which reduce cerebral oedema improve the patient's long-term outlook (Study Group, 1977).

In the established stroke there is some evidence that betahistine modestly improves some but not all cerebral functions (Pathy *et al.*, 1977). Similar studies using cerebral vasodilators have been inconclusive.

NARCOTIC ANALGESICS

The perception of pain follows a definite pathway (see Table 3.14). The mode of action of narcotic analgesics is in part through receptor sites in the brain and elsewhere. Within the body natural 'opiate-like' substances—endorphins and enkephalins—occur (Hughes and Kosterlitz, 1977). There is probably more than one receptor, or the receptor may exist in more than one state. Martin *et al.* (1976) postulated three types of receptor to explain the range of action of the narcotic analgesics.

Table 3.14   Pain-perception pathway

Sensory ganglia ↓ Substantia gelatinosa in the posterior grey horn of the spinal cord ↓ Lateral spinothalamic tract ↓ Ventroposterior and intralaminar nuclei of the thalamus

Table 3.15   Narcotic analgesics

Group A: Naturally occurring—morphine

Group B: Synthetic
    (1) 5-ring—diamorphine
    (2) 4-ring—morphinans—levorphanol
    (3) 3-ring—benzmorphans—phenazocine, pentazocine
    (4) Pethidine
    (5) Methadone

Table 3.15 shows the various subgroups. The narcotic analgesics are metabolized in the liver. Changes in hepatic blood flow can greatly influence their metabolism (Blaschke, 1977). Morphine, pethidine, and pentazocine are subject to hepatic first-pass metabolism. This renders their bioavailability low after oral dosage.

The doses of all drugs in this group need to be tailored to individual needs due to the individual differences in availability, elimination, and the great variation in the perception of pain. The elderly are particularly sensitive to the depressant effects of narcotic analgesics and experience more analgesia for a given dose of analgesic than younger subjects (Belville *et al.*, 1971). The plasma concentrations of morphine and pethidine have also been shown to be raised in elderly subjects (Berkowitz, 1976; Mather and Meffin, 1978).

Narcotic analgesics delay gastric emptying very markedly and thus can alter the absorption of concomitantly administered oral drugs. They also decrease intestinal secretions: constipation from diminished intestinal motility can be particularly troublesome.

The indications for their use do not differ from those of younger subjects. Table 3.16 gives suggested doses for the various drugs in elderly subjects. A recent survey (Caradoc-Davies, 1981) illustrated the increased likelihood of opiate toxicity in the elderly unless smaller than 'normal' doses are used. This study recommended that opiates should only be given intravenously. It also found nausea to be a relatively rare complication. Adverse effects on respiratory function were reversed by naloxone. The hypotension and bradycardia associated with opiate toxicity responded to elevation of the legs. Atropine was rarely needed.

Table 3.16   Narcotic analgesics

Drug	Dose	Points
(1) Pentazocine		Should be avoided in the elderly
(2) Morphine	5–10 mg	Severe pain
(3) Buprenorphine	300–600 mg i.m. four times daily or 200–400 mg sublingually four times daily	
(4) Dextromoramide	5–20 mg four times daily	
(5) Diamorphine	2.5 mg 4-hourly	Severe pain
(6) Dipipanone	10–30 mg 4-hourly	
(7) Levorphanol	1.5–4.5 mg b.d.	Longer lasting
(8) Papaveretum	10–20 mg	

If these drugs are being used to control terminal pain then 'Brompton mixture' may well be the most suitable preparation.

Nausea can be controlled by sparine.

Pain should not be allowed to surface—once the fear of pain has been removed it is not infrequently found that the dose of these drugs can be reduced.

The St Christopher's Hospice schedule should be used.

EPILEPSY

Much has been written about epilepsy in elderly subjects, in the main from highly specialized neurological centres. The more ordinary presentation in a general geriatric unit has been detailed by Hildick-Smith (1974). Of the 50 patients in her survey 21 cases were due to cerebrovascular disease and 7 due to dementia. Neoplasm, either primary or secondary, accounted for only 5 cases. Seven cases were thought to be idiopathic and only 5 cases had a potentially remediable cause (metabolic upset and heart block).

84

Late-onset idiopathic epilepsy is relatively common. It responds well to conventional anticonvulsant therapy. In a significant number of cases the fits are exclusively noctural.

It is, however, important to exclude reversible and treatable causes. The vigour with which investigations should be pursued must be in part governed by the general state of the patient. There is no point in resorting to elaborate neurological investigations in a patient who would be totally unfit to withstand craniotomy.

In most cases a detailed history of the onset and nature of the fits accompanied by some easily obtained non-invasive investigations will be adequate. These should include ECG to exclude cardiac causes of 'fits', e.g. Stokes–Adams attacks, biochemical screen to exclude metabolic causes, chest and skull X-ray to exclude obvious tumours, EEG, and isotope brain scan.

In patients over 60 years the majority of tumours causing epilepsy are malignant. However, as age advances the overall incidence of tumours declines. Good claims have been made for the diagnostic accuracy of the combination of EEG and isotope brain scan (Decker and Knott, 1972; Gilday and Reba, 1972). However, the interpretation of the EEG in the elderly requires a great degree of skill. At the best of times there are numerous 'abnormalities' which may occur in a 'normal' EEG with age. The main finding in the EEG which has diagnostic significance in the elderly is a focus of slow delta activity.

Isotope brain scanning is useful because if multiple tumour deposits are detected the relatives can be advised accordingly, the patient spared further investigation and appropriate care arranged. If the patient has a lesion detected by scanning, and is otherwise fit and healthy, the decision to proceed further can only be taken in consultation with a neurosurgeon.

The basic classification of seizures does not change with age: Generalized, Partial, Unilateral, and Unclassified (Gastaut, 1970). The drug therapy is in the main governed by the nature of the seizures. All the anticonvulsants act by depressing neuronal excitability by stabilizing cell membranes, and preventing the spread of seizures by modifying synaptic transmission. Nearly all the anticonvulsant drugs are cumulative. It is important that blood levels be regularly estimated.

The anticonvulsant drugs, doses, and clinical indications are detailed in Table 3.17. Table 3.18 lists their side-effects. Table 3.19 gives a list of clinically important drug interactions.

The only anticonvulsant to be extensively studied in the elderly is phenytoin. The plasma levels show an increase with age (Houghton *et*

Table 3.17 Antiepileptic drugs—doses and uses

Drug	Dose (mg)	Therapeutic levels (μg/ml)	Seizure type	$T_{1/2}$ (h)	Points
Phenobarbitone	60–400	10–30	Tonic/clonic Psychomotor	48–120	
Sodium valproate	600–2000	40–120	Tonic/clonic Psychomotor Akinetic/myoclonic	13–21	
Phenytoin	200–600	10–20	Tonic/clonic Psychomotor	20–30	Increase dose slowly; use only *one* brand
Carbamazipine	400–1600	4–12	Tonic/clonic Psychomotor	10–20	

Status epilepticus—diazepam:
5 mg/min by slow i.v. injection, up to total of 0.25 mg/kg. If ineffective, paraldehyde 5–10 ml i.m.; or chlormethiazole 0.8% i.v. infusion, 40–100 ml at 3–10 ml/min.

Table 3.18 Side-effects of antiepileptic drugs

Phenobarbitone—see barbiturates

Phenytoin	Nausea, vomiting
	Confusion
	Dizziness, headache
	Tremor
	Insomnia
	Ataxia
	Slurred speech ⎫
	Nystagmus ⎬ Overdose
	Hirsutes ⎭
	Acne
	Gingival hypertrophy
	SLE
	Hepatitis
	Megaloblastic anaemia
Sodium valproate	Nausea
	Hair loss
	Oedema
	Impaired liver function → hepatic failure
	Thrombocytopenia

Table 3.18   Continued

Carbamazepine	Dizziness
	Drowsiness
	Upset vision
	Leucopenia
	Skin rash
	Nausea and vomiting

Table 3.19   Clinically important drug interactions with antiepileptic drugs

Phenobarbitone	Sulthiame increases phenobarbitone levels
	Sodium valproate increases phenobarbitone levels
Sodium valproate	Phenytoin may reduce valproate levels
Phenytoin	Chloramphenicol increases phenytoin levels
	Dicoumarol increases phenytoin levels
	Disulfiram increases phenytoin levels
	Isoniazid increases phenytoin levels
	Phenylbutazone increases phenytoin levels
	Sulphonamides increase phenytoin levels
	Carbamazepine reduces phenytoin levels
Carbamazepine	Dextropropoxyphene increases carbamazepine levels
	Phenobarbitone decreases carbamazepine levels

al., 1975). Total plasma clearance increases with age due to a decrease in plasma binding (Hooper *et al.*, 1974). Hayes *et al.* (1975) showed that this change was secondary to an age-dependent decrease in plasma albumin.

If care is used there should be no significant problems treating epilepsy in the elderly.

ANTIPSYCHOTIC DRUGS

This drug group comprises neuroleptics and major tranquillizers—phenothiazines, butyrophenones, thioxanthines, tetrabenazine.

They are used to treat psychoses and severe confusional states in the elderly such as agitated dementia (Silverman, 1977). They act mainly on the hypothalamus and the reticular activating system. Unfortunately, they have a great propensity to produce extrapyramidal side-effects in the elderly.

There are three main groups in the phenothiazine family:

Group 1: aliphatic side-chain derivatives:
        chlorpromazine
        promazine
Group 2: piperazine derivatives:
        fluphenazine
        perphenazine
        trifluoperazine
        thiethylperazine
        thiorpropazate hydrochloride
Group 3: piperadine derivatives:
        thioridazine
        pericyazine

All these drugs block cholinergic, dopaminergic, and triptaminergic receptors. Drugs in Groups 1 and 2 are strong α-blockers and weak anti-cholinergics, whilst for those in Group 3 these clinical properties are reversed.

The two most commonly used members of this group are chlor-promazine and thioridazine. Haloperidol can also be useful in the elderly in the management of severely agitated hyperactive psychotic states. However, side-effects severely limit its long-term use.

The bioavailability of chlorpromazine may be reduced by delayed gastric emptying or by drugs which reduce intestinal motility (Rivera-Calimlin, 1978). The bioavailability is also variable (27–67%) due to metabolism in the gut wall (Dahl and Strandgord, 1977). It is highly lipid-soluble and extensively protein-bound.

Axelsson and Martensson (1976) found that the plasma concentrations of thioridazine were, for any given dose, higher in older than younger subjects.

There are several points to remember about the use of these drugs in the elderly:

(1) Extrapyramidal side-effects are common (Salzman *et al.*, 1976). Although they are relatively easy to detect it is difficult to predict which patients will develop them as they depend on the particular drug, the dose, and the susceptibility of the patient. Dystonia may appear after only a few doses, whereas the Parkinsonian picture takes longer to develop (Ayd, 1961).

    Tardive dyskinesia is a severe and usually irreversible and untreat-able side-effect (Editorial, 1979). It occurs in patients on long-term therapy. Such patients must be reviewed regularly.

(2) Postural hypotension is common with these preparations in the elderly. Routine measurements of blood pressure must be part of the surveillance programme of patients receiving these drugs.

(3) These drugs also interfere with temperature regulation, increasing the risk of hypothermia in the old. The suggested drugs and initial doses are detailed in Table 3.20, and their side-effects in Table 3.21.

These drugs need to be used with extreme caution in the elderly. A precise diagnosis is required. All other causes such as an underlying medical condition or drug reaction must be excluded. Raskind *et al.* (1976) found

Table 3.20   Suggested initial doses of antipsychotic drugs

Chlorpromazine	10–25 mg t.d.s.
Thioridazine	10 mg t.d.s., up to maximum of 100 mg per day
Haloperidol	0.5–1.5 mg t.d.s.

These doses should be increased slowly.

Table 3.21   Side-effects of antipsychotic drugs

Chlorpromazine	Extrapyramidal symptoms
	Hypothermia
	Occasionally causes hyperpyrexia
	Drowsiness, apathy
	Nightmares
	Agitation
	Dry mouth, blurred vision
	Difficulty in micturition
	Hypotension
	Cardiac arrhythmias
	Blood dyscrasias
	Photosensitivity/skin rashes
	Jaundice
	Corneal opacities
	Nodules at injection sites
Thioridazine	As above—less sedation and fewer extrapyramidal effects
	Likely to cause hypotension
	Pigmentary retionopathy
Haloperidol	As above—less sedation than chlorpromazine but more frequent extrapyramidal effects
	Occasionally causes tardive dyskinesia
	Blood dyscrasias

that 25% of apparently 'psychiatric' elderly patients had an undiagnosed medical illness as the root of the problem (CCF, hyperthyroidism, diabetes, etc.).

Drugs such as these must never be used as a solution to social problems, as illustrated by a cautionary tale from Nottingham:

> An old lady of 90 years, rather argumentative and domineering, had persuaded her son, daughter-in-law, and grandchildren to move into her house with her. There was considerable friction among the three generations. The family practitioner was summoned and prescribed 50 mg chlorpromazine as required. Every time the old lady opened her mouth to complain she had 50 mg chlorpromazine slipped in. In the end she became confused, unable to walk, and doubly incontinent. An application for long-term care was made. However, on stopping the chlorpromazine the old lady recovered fully. By some sleight of hand with social services and housing departments, all lived happily and separately ever after.

REFERENCES AND BIBLIOGRAPHY

Adam, K. *et al.* (1976) Nitrazepam: lastingly effective but trouble on withdrawal. *Brit. Med. J.*, **1**, 1558–60.

Alexanderson, B. *et al.* (1969) Steady state plasma levels on nortriptyline in twins: influence of genetic factors and drug therapy. *Brit. Med. J.*, **4**, 764–8.

Alexanderson, B. (1973) Prediction of steady state plasma levels of nortriptyline from single oral dose kinetics: a study in twins. *Eur. J. Clin. Pharmac.*, **6**, 44–53.

Amdisen, A. (1977) Serum monitoring and clinical pharmacokinetics of lithium. *Clin. Pharmacokinetics*, **2**, 73.

Asberg, M. (1974a) Individualisation of treatment with tricyclic compounds. *Med. Clin. N. Am.*, **58**, 1083–91.

Asberg, M. (1974b) Plasma nortriptyline levels and clinical effects. *Clin. Pharmac. Ther.*, **16**, 215–29.

Asberg, M. *et al.* (1971) Relationship between plasma level and therapeutic effect of nortriptyline. *Brit. Med. J.*, **3**, 331–4.

Ashcroft, G. W. (1975) Management of depression. *Brit. Med. J.*, **2**, 372.

Axelrod, J. (1971) Noradrenaline fate and control of its biosynthesis. *Science*, **173**, 598.

Axelsson, R. and Martensson, E. (1976) Serum concentration and elimination from serum of thioridozine in psychiatric patients. *Current Ther. Res.*, **19**, 242.

Ayd, F. J. (1961) A survey of drug-induced extrapyramidal reactions. *JAMA*, **175**, 102–8.

Baldaressini, R. J. (1975) The basis for amine hypothesis in affective disorders. *Arch. Gen. Psych.*, **32**, 1087.

Barbeau, A. (1973) Treatment of Parkinson's disease with L-dopa and Ro 4–4602: Review and present status. *Adv. Neurol.*, **2**, 173.

Barbeau, A. (1975) Long-term assessment of levodopa in Parkinson's disease. *Can. Med. Assoc. J.*, **112**, 1379.

Beckman, H. and Goodwin, F. K. (1975) Antidepressant response to tricyclics and urinary MHPG. *Arch. Gen. Psych.*, **32**, 17.

Belville, J. W. *et al.* (1971) Influence of age on pain relief from analgesics. *JAMA*, **217**, 1835.

Berkowitz, B. A. (1976) The relation of pharmacokinetics to pharmacological activity: morphine, methadone and naloxone. *Clin. Pharmacokinetics*, **1**, 219.

Bernheimer, H. *et al.* (1965) *Zur Differenzierung des Parkinson-Syndroms*. 8th International Congress of Neurology (Vienna Medical Academy).

Bianchine, J. D. and Shaw, G. M. (1976) Clinical pharmacokinetics of levodopa in Parkinson's disease. *Clin. Pharmacokinetics*, **1**, 313.

Birkmayer, H. and Hornykiewicz, O. (1961) Der L-3, 4 dioxyphenylalanin Effeckt bei der Parkinsonakinese. *Wien Klin. Wochenschr.*, **73**, 787.

Blaschke, T. F. (1977) Protein binding and kinetics of drugs in liver disease. *Clin. Pharmacokinetics*, **2**, 32.

Bond, A. J. and Lader, M. H. (1972) Residual effects of hypnotics. *Psychopharmacologia*, **25**, 117–32.

Boston Collaborative Drug Surveillance Programme (1973) Clinical depression of the central nervous system due to diazepam and chlordiazepoxide: relation to cigarette smoking and age. *New Engl. J. Med.*, **288**, 277–80.

Bowen, D. M. and Davison, A. N. (1978) Biochemical changes in the normal ageing brain. In B. Isaacs (ed.), *Recent Advances in Geriatric Medicine*. Churchill Livingstone, Edinburgh, London, and New York.

Braithwaite, R. A. *et al.*(1972) Plasma concentrations of amitriptyline and clinical response. *Lancet*, **1**, 1297–300.

Braithwaite, R. A. *et al.* (1978) The pharmacokinetics of nortriptyline in patients with high plasma levels. *Clin. Pharmac. Ther.*, **23**, 303–8.

Brewis, M. *et al.* (1962) Neurological disease in an English city. *Acta. Neurol. Scand.*, **24** (suppl.), 42; 31.

Briggs, R. S. *et al.* (1980) Improved hypnotic treatment using chlormethiazole and temazepam. *Brit. Med. J.*, **1**, 601–4.

Broe, G. A. and Caird, F. I. (1973) Levodopa for Parkinsonism in elderly and demented patients. *Med. J. Aust.*, **1**, 630.

Brogden, R. N. *et al.* (1971) Levodopa: a review of its pharmacological properties and therapeutic uses. *Drugs*, **2**, 262.

Brogden, R. N. *et al.* (1978) Mianserin: a review. *Drugs*, **16**, 27.

Calne, D. B. (1977) Developments in the pharmacology and therapeutics of Parkinsonism. *Ann. Neurol.*, **1**, 111.

Calne, D. B. *et al.* (1978) Long-term treatment of Parkinson's disease with bromocriptine. *Lancet*, **1**, 735.

Caradoc-Davies, T. H. (1981) Opiate toxicity in elderly patients. *Brit. Med. J.*, **283**, 907–8.

Carlsson, A. *et al.* (1969) Effects of antidepressant drugs on the depletion of intraneuronal brain catecholamines. *Eur. J. Pharmacol.*, **5**, 367.

Castleden, C. M. *et al.* (1977) Increased sensitivity to nitrazepam in old age. *Brit. Med. J.*, **1**, 10–12.

Chase, T. N. *et al.* (1976) Clinical and pharmacological studies of the 'on-off' phenomenon. In Birkmeyer, H. and Hornykiewicz, O. (eds) *Advances in Parkinsonism*. Editiones Roches, Basel.

Clarke, G. F. M. (1904) A case of veronal poisoning. *Lancet*, **1**, 223.

Dahl, S. G. and Strandgord, R. E. (1977) Pharmacokinetics of chlorpromazine after single and chronic dosage. *Clin. Pharmacol. Ther.*, **21**, 437.

Decker, D. A. Jr. and Knott, J. R. (1972) The EEG in intrinsic supratentorial brain tumours: a comparative evaluation. *Electroenceph. Clin. Neurophysiol.*, **33**, 303–10.

Desjacques, P. *et al.* (1973) Effets cardiovasculaire de la L-dopa et de l'inhibiteur de la decarboxylase chez Parkinsons. *Schweiz. Med. Wochenschr.*, **103**, 1783.

Diaz-Guerro, R. *et al.* (1946) The sleep of patients with manic depressive psychosis. *Psychosom. Med.*, **8**, 399.

Duvoisin, R. C. (1969) In Crane, G. E. and Gardiner, R. J. (eds), *Psychotropic Drugs and Dysfunction of the Basal Ganglia*, p. 34. US Public Health Services, Washington.

Editorial (1974) The management of elderly demented patients. *Brit. Med. J.*, **1**, 1301.

Editorial (1979) Tardive dyskinesia. *Lancet*, **2**, 447.

Editorial (1981) Levodopa—long-term impact on Parkinson's disease. *Brit. Med. J.*, **282**, 417–18.

Ehringer, H. and Hornykiewicz, O. (1960) Verteilung von Noradrenalin und Dopamin in Genurn des Menschen und ihe Verhalten bei Erkrangungen des extrapyramidalen Systems. *Klin. Wochenschr.*, **38**, 1236.

Evans, G. J. and Jarvis, E. H. (1972) Nitrazepam in the elderly. *Brit. Med. J.*, **2**, 487.

Exton-Smith, A. N. (1967) The use and abuse of hypnotics. *Gerontol. Clinica*, **9**, 264–9.

Exton-Smith, A. N. and Maclean, I. (1979) Uses and abuses of chlormethiazole. *Lancet*, **1**, 1093.

Exton-Smith, A. N. and Witts, D. J. (1979) A comparison of chlormethiazole and nitrazepam as hypnotics in elderly subjects. *Current Trends in Therapeutics*, pp. 39–47. MES, Oxford.

Feigenson, J. S. *et al.* (1976) Piribedil: synergistic effect in multi-drug regimens for Parkinsonism. *Neurology*, **26**, 430.

Flamm, E. S. *et al.* (1975) Phosphodiesterase inhibitors and cerebral vasospasms. *Arch Neurol.*, **32**, 569.

Flood, M. K. (1979) Pyritinol hydrochloride and senile dementia. *Brit. Med. J.*, **1**, 1148.

Forrester, T. *et al.* (1975) Vascular and metabolic effects of systemic A.T.P. on the cerebral circulation. In Harper,   ., Jennett,   ., Miller,   ., and Rowan,   . (eds), *Blood Flow and Metabolism in the Brain*. Churchill-Livingstone, Edinburgh and London.

Friis, M. L. *et al.* (1979) Transfer of bromocriptine across the blood–brain barrier in man. *Acta Neurol. Scand.*, **59**, 88–95.

Garland, H. G. (1952) Parkinsonism. *Brit. Med. J.*, **1**, 153.

Gastaut, H. (1970) Clinical and electroencephalographic classification of seizures. *Epilepsia*, **1**, 102.

Gedye, J. L. *et al.* (1972) A method for measuring mental performance in the elderly and its use in a pilot trial of meclofenoxate in dementia. *Age and Ageing*, **1**, 74–80.

Gibson, I. I. J. M. (1966) Barbiturate delirium. *Practitioner*, **197**, 345.

Gilday, D. L. and Reba, R. C. (1972) The role of brain scanning in the differential diagnosis of seizure. *Can. Med. Assoc. J.*, **106**, 1091–4.

Glen, A. I. M. (1980) The pharmacology of dementia. *Hospital Update*, **6**, 977–87.

Goldstein, S. E. *et al.* (1978) Comparison of oxazepam, flurazepam and chloral hydrate as hypnotic sedatives in geriatric patients. *J. Am. Geriat. Soc.*, **24**, 366–71.

Goodman, L. S. and Gilman, A. (1980) *The Pharmacological Basis of Therapeutics*. Baillière & Tindall, London.

Greenblatt, D. J. and Shader, R. I. (1974) Drug therapy. *New Engl. J. Med.*, **291**, 1239.

Greenblatt, D. J. *et al.* (1975) Pharmacokinetics in clinical medicine. *Dis. Nerv. Syst.*, **36**, 6.

Greenblatt, D. J. *et al.* (1977) Toxicity of high dose flurazepam in the elderly. *Clin. Pharmacol. Ther.*, **21**, 355–61.

Gudmundsson, K. R. (1967) A clinical survey of Parkinsonism in Iceland. *Acta Neurol. Scand.*, **33** (suppl.), 43.

Hall, M. R. P. (1975) Use of drugs in the elderly. *N.Y. State J. Med.*, **3**, 67–72.

Hammer, W. and Sjøqvist, F. (1967) Plasma levels of monomethylated tricyclic antidepressant during treatment with imipromine-like compounds. *Life Sci.*, **6**, 1895–1903.

Hayes, M. J. *et al.* (1975) Changes in drug metabolism with age: phenytoin clearance and protein binding. *Brit. J. Clin. Pharmacol.*, **2**, 69–72.

Hewick, D. S. *et al.* (1977) Age as a factor affecting lithium therapy. *Brit. J. Clin. Pharmacol.*, **4**, 201.

Hildick-Smith, M. (1974) Epilepsy in the elderly. *Age and Ageing*, **3**, 203.

Hoehn, M. M. and Yahr, M. D. (1967) Parkinsonism: onset, progression and mortality. *Neurology*, **17**, 427–42.

Hollister, L. E. *et al.* (1967) Specific therapy in newly admitted schizophrenics. *Clin. Pharmacol. Ther.*, **11**, 49.

Hooper, W. D. *et al.* (1974) Plasma protein binding of diphenylhydantoin: effect of sex hormones, renal and hepatic disease. *Clin. Pharmacol. Ther.*, **15**, 276–82.

Houghton, G. W. *et al.* (1975) Effect of age, sex, height and weight on serum phenytoin concentrations. *Br. J. Clin. Pharmacol.*, **2**, 251–6.

Hughes, J. and Kosterlitz, H. W. (1977) Opioid peptides. *Brit. Med. Bull.*, **33**, 157.

Hughes, R. C. *et al.* (1971) Levodopa in Parkinsonism: the effect of withdrawal of anticholinergic drugs. *Brit. Med. J.*, **2**, 487.

Hunter, K. R. *et al.* (1973) Sustained levodopa therapy in Parkinsonism. *Lancet*, **2**, 929–31.

Isbell, H. (1950) Barbiturate withdrawal. *Ann. Intern. Med.*, **33**, 108.

Johnson, W. C. (1975) A neglected modality in psychiatric treatment—the M.A.O.I. *Dis. Nerv. System*, **36**, 521.

Karim, A. K. B. M. and Price-Evans, D. A. (1976) Polymorphic acetylation of nitrazepam. *J. Med. Genet.*, **13**, 17.

Kartzinel, R. and Calne, D. B. (1976) Studies with bromocriptine. I. On–off phenomena. *Neurol. Minneap.*, **26**, 508–10.

Kebabian, J. N. and Calne, D. B. (1979). Multiple receptors for dopamine. *Nature (London)*, **277**, 93–6.

Klotz, U. *et al.* (1975) The effects of age and liver disease on the disposition and elimination of diazepam in the adult man. *J. Clin. Invest.*, **55**, 347–59.

Kragh-Sørensen, P. *et al.* (1973) Plasma nortriptyline levels in endogenous depression. *Lancet*, **1**, 113–15

Kragh-Sørensen, P. *et al.* (1976) Self-inhibiting action of nortriptyline's anti-depressant effect at high plasma levels. *Psychopharmacologia*, **45**, 305–16.

Kurland, L. T. (1958) In W. S. Fields (ed.), *Pathogenesis and Treatment of Parkinsonism*. Thomas, Springfield, Ill.

Learoyd, B. M. (1972) Psychotropic drugs and the elderly patient. *Med. J. Aust.*, **1**, 1131–3.

Lees, A. J. and Stern, G. M. (1981) Sustained bromocriptine therapy in previously untreated patients with Parkinson's disease. *Res. Clin. Forums*, **3** (2), 29–32.

Lehmann, K. and Merten, K. (1974) Elimination of lithium dependent on age in healthy people and those with renal insufficiency. *Int. J. Clin. Pharmacol. Ther. Toxicol.*, **10**, 292.

Lewis, C. *et al.* (1978) Trial of levodopa in senile dementia. *Brit. Med. J.*, **1**, 550.

Lipani, J. A. (1978) Preference study of the hypnotic efficacy of triazolam 0.125 mg compared to placebo in geriatric patients with insomnia. *Curr. Ther. Res.*, **24**, 397–402.

Lloyd-Evans, S. *et al.* (1978) Assessment of drug therapy in chronic brain failure. *Gerontology*, **24**, 304–11.

Macdonald, J. B. and Macdonald, E. T. (1977) Nocturnal femoral fracture and continuing widespread use of barbiturate hypnotics. *Brit. Med. J.*, **2**, 483–5.

McDowell, F. H. and Sweet, R. D. (1976) In Birkmayer, H. and Hornykiewicz, O. (eds) *Advances in Parkinsonism*, p. 603. Editiones-Roche, Basel.

McIlwain, H. (1977) Extended roles in the brain for second messenger systems. *Neuroscience*, **2**, 357.

Maas, J. W. (1975) Biogenic amines and depression. *Arch. Gen. Psychiatry*, **32**, 1357.

Mars, H. and Krall, J. (1971) L-dopa and cardiac arrhythmias. *New Engl. J. Med.*, **285**, 1437.

Marsden, C. D. and Parkes, J. D. (1976) On–off effects in patients with Parkinsonism on chronic levodopa therapy. *Lancet*, **1**, 292.

Martin, W. R. *et al.* (1976) The effects of morphine and nalorphine-like drugs on dependent and non-dependent dogs. *J. Pharmacol. Exp. Ther.*, **197**, 517.

Mason, R. W. *et al.* (1978) Pharmacokinetics of lithium. *Clin. Pharmacokinetics*, **3**, 241.

Mather, L. E. and Meffin, P. J. (1978) Clinical pharmacokinetics of pethidine. *Clin. Pharmacokinetics*, **3**, 352.

Mellstrom, B. and Tybring, G. (1977) Ion-part liquid chromatography of steady state plasma levels of chlomopromine and desmethylchlomipromine. *J. Chromatog. Bio-med. Appl.*, **143**, 597–605.

Metzler, C. M. *et al.* (1977) Bioavailability and pharmacokinetics of orally administered triazolam in normal subjects. *Clin. Pharmacol. Ther.*, **21**, 111–12.

Meynaud, A. *et al.* (1975) Effet du naphtidropuryl sur le métabolisme énergétique cérébral chez la souris. *Thérapie*, **30**, 777.

Montgomery, S. *et al.* (1978) High plasma levels of nortriptyline in the treatment of depression. *Clin. Pharmacol. Ther.*, **23**, 309–14.

Moody, J. P. and Tait, S. (1967) Plasma levels of imipramine and desmethylimipramine during therapy. *Brit. J. Psychiatry*, **113**, 183–93.

Moore, R. G. *et al.* (1975) Pharmacokinetics of chlormethiazole in humans. *Eur. J. Clin. Pharmacol.*, **8**, 353–7.

Mulley, G. *et al.* (1978) Dexamethasone in acute stroke. *Brit. Med. J.*, **2**, 994.

Nation, R. L. *et al.* (1976) Pharmacokinetics of chlormethiazole following intravenous administration in the elderly. *Eur. J. Clin. Pharmacol.*, **10**, 407–15.

Nies, A. *et al.* (1977) Relationship between age and tricyclic antidepressant levels. *Am. J. Psychiatry*, **134**, 790.

Oswald, I. *et al.* (1972) On the slowness of action of tricyclic antidepressants. *Brit. J. Psychiatry*, **120**, 673.

Parkes, J. D. (1979) Bromocriptine in the treatment of Parkinsonism. *Drugs*, **17**, 365.

Parkes, J. D. *et al.* (1971) Treatment of Parkinson's disease with amantadine and levodopa. *Lancet*, **1**, 1183.

Parkinson, J. (1817) *An Essay on the Shaking Palsy*. Sherwood, Neely and Jones, London.

Pathy, J. *et al.* (1977) Betahistine hydrochloride (Serc) in cerebrovascular disease: a placebo-controlled study. *Age and Ageing*, **6**, 179–84.

Pathy, M. S. (1977) A comparison of 2 sedative–hypnotic drugs. *Age and Ageing*, **6**, 91–4.

Pearce, J. M. S. (1978) Aetiology and natural history of Parkinson's disease. *Brit. Med. J.*, **4**, 1664.

Pinder, R. M. *et al.* (1977) Doxepin up-to-date. *Drugs*, **13**, 161.

Pollock, M. and Hornabrook, R. W. (1966) The prevalence, natural history and dementia of Parkinson's disease. *Brain*, **89**, 429–48.

Raskind, M. A. *et al.* (1976) Helping the elderly psychiatric patient in crisis. *Geriatrics*, **31**, 51–6.

Reavill, C., Jenner, P., and Marsden, C. D. (1981) Pharmacological and biochemical aspects of the mechanism of bromocriptine. *Res. and Clin. Forums*, **3** (2), 7–17.

Reisdenberg, M. M. (1978) Relationship between diazepam, dose, plasma level, age and CNS depression. *Clin. Pharmacol. Ther.*, **23**, 371–4.

Rinne, U. K. *et al.* (1973) Brain acetylcholinesterase in Parkinson's disease. *Acta Neurol. Scand.*, **49**, 215.

Rivera-Calimlin, L. *et al.* (1978) Effect of lithium on plasma chlorpromazine levels. *Clin. Pharmacol. Ther.*, **23**, 451.

Robinson, D. S. *et al.* (1978) Clinical pharmacology of phenelzine. *Arch. Gen. Psychiatry*, **35**, 629–35.

Salzman, C. *et al.* (1976) Clinical psychopharmacology and the elderly patient. *N.Y. State J. Med.*, **76**, 71–7.

Sanford, J. R. A. (1975) Tolerance of debility in elderly dependants by supporters at home: its significance for hospital practice. *Brit. Med. J.*, **3**, 471–3.

Schildkraut, J. J. (1974) The current status of classifying depressive illness. *Psychopharmacol. Bull.*, **10**, 5.

Schwab, R. S. *et al.* (1969) Amantadine in the treatment of Parkinson's disease. *JAMA*, **208**, 1168.

Scott, S. and Caird, F. I. (1981) Speech therapy for patients with Parkinson's disease. *Br. Med. J.*, **283**, 1088.

Shaw, K. M., Lees, A. J., and Stern, G. M. (1980) The impact of treatment with levodopa on Parkinson's disease. *Q.J. Med.*, **49**, 283–93.

Silverman, G. (1977) Management of the elderly agitated demented patient. *Brit. Med. J.*, **2**, 318.

Sjøqvist, F. *et al.* (1969) Pharmacological significance of plasma levels of antidepressants. *Excerpta Medica Int. Congr. Ser.*, **180**, 128–36.

Sjøqvist, F. (1975) Assessment of antidepressants. In Breckenridge, A. (ed.), *Advanced Medicine Topics*. Pitman, Tunbridge Wells.

Snider, S. R. *et al.* (1976) Correlation of behavioural inhibition or excitation produced by bromocriptine with changes in brain catecholamine turnover. *J. Pharm. Pharmacol.*, **28**, 563–6.

Snyder, S. H. (1977) Opiate receptors and internal opiates. *Sci. Am.*, **236**, 44–56.

Squires, R. F. and Braestrup, C. (1977) Benzodiazepine receptors in the rat brain. *Nature*, **266**, 732–4.

Stromberg, U. *et al.* (1970) On the mode of action of amantadine. *J. Pharm. Pharmacol.*, **22**, 959.

Study Group, Joint Committee for Stroke Resources (1977) Brain, edema and stroke. *Stroke*, **8**, 512.

Sutcliffe, R. L. G. (1973) L-dopa therapy in elderly patients with Parkinson's disease. *Age and Ageing*, **2**, 34.

Sweet, R. D. and McDowell, F. H. (1975). Five years treatment of Parkinson's disease with levodopa; therapeutic results and survival of 100 patients. *Ann. Int. Med.*, **83**, 456.

Teychenne, P. F. *et al.* (1981) Low dose bromocriptine therapy in Parkinson's disease. *Res. and Clin. Forums*, **3** (2), 37–47.

Triggs, E. J. and Nation, R. L. (1975) Pharmacokinetics in the aged: a review. *J. Pharmacokin. Biopharmacol.*, **3**, 387–418.

Vignalou. J. and Beck, H. (1973) La L-dopa chez 122 Parkinsonien de plus de 70 ans. *Gerontol. Clin.*, **15**, 50.

Weil-Malherbe, H. and Szara, S. I. (1971) *The Biochemistry of Functional and Experimental Psychoses*, p. 55. Thomas, Springfield, Ill.

Wells, F. O. (1973) Prescribing barbiturates: drug substitution in general practice. *J. Roy. Coll. Gen. Pract.*, **23**, 164–7.

White, S. F. (1976) Plasma concentrations of antidepressants and clinical effects in depressed women. *Brit. J. Psychiatry*, **128**, 384-90.

Wilkinson, G. R. and Shand, D. G. (1975) A physiological approach to hepatic drug clearance. *Clin. Pharmacol. Ther.*, **18**, 377–90.

Wilkinson, G. R. (1979) In Crooks, J. and Stevenson, I. H. (eds.) *Drugs and the Elderly*, p. 109. Macmillan, London.
Williamson, J. (1978) Depression in the elderly. *Age and Ageing*, **7** (suppl. 35).
Wulff, M. H. (1959) The barbiturate withdrawal syndrome. *Electroencephalography and Clinical Neurophysiology*, Suppl. No. 14.
Yahr, M. D. *et al.* (1971) Modification of levodopa therapy of Parkinsonism by α-methyl-dopa-hydrazine. *Trans. Am. Neurol. Ass.*, **96**, 55.
Yesavage, J. A. *et al.* (1979) Vasodilators in senile dementias. *Arch. Gen. Psychiatry*, **36**, 220–3.
Zeigler, V. E. *et al.* (1976) Nortriptyline levels and therapeutic response. *Clin. Pharmacol. Ther.*, **19**, 795–801.

Chapter 4

Drugs acting on the cardiovascular system

Many aspects of therapy in the elderly are controversial, but the treatment of cardiovascular disease is a medical minefield. For instance, when does elevated blood pressure become hypertension? Does hypertension in the elderly matter? If therapy is indicated, how low do you hope to get the blood pressure? Do patients need maintenance digoxin? Do patients on diuretics require potassium supplements? These problems are of great importance, since digoxin and antihypertensives are among the greatest culprits in causing adverse drug reactions.

DRUGS IN THE TREATMENT OF HYPERTENSION

Many epidemiological studies have been carried out on the impact of hypertension, but the elderly are conspicuously absent from the subjects studied. Controlled therapeutic trials have been particularly careful to exclude the elderly. Indeed, one major study discontinued follow-up after the age of 70 years on the grounds of advanced age precluding any therapeutic benefit. The only studies so far directed specifically at the elderly are those of Macfarlane and Kennedy (1973), Eisalo *et al.* (1974), and Lundborg and Steen (1976). Much has been written on the subject, but tragically the reports tend to be anecdotal or dogma based on opinion rather than fact.

High blood pressure is common in the elderly, affecting women more than men (Hamilton *et al.*, 1954), but what is its prevalence? This is greatly influenced by what you define as the upper limit of normal (Alderman and Yano, 1976) and by how measurements are made (Carey *et al.*, 1976). Studies have varied widely in their definition of the upper limit of normal systolic pressure from 130 to 200 mm Hg and diastolic pressure from 90 to 120 mm Hg. These levels are entirely arbitrary. The Framingham study (Kannel and Gordon, 1974) defined hypertension as systolic pressure greater than 160 mm Hg and diastolic pressure greater than 95 mm Hg. On such levels some 30% of men between 65 and 74 years entering the study were hypertensive. Others have claimed that

65% of 70-year-old men are hypertensive (Master, 1952; Chrysant *et al.*, 1976).

Systolic and diastolic pressure have long been known to increase with age. This change occurs in both sexes. The systolic pressure tends to rise more than the diastolic pressure (Society of Actuaries, 1959; Master and Laser, 1961; United States National Centre for Health Statistics, 1977). Because this change is so common in the aged in Western cultures it has unfortunately become accepted as normal. But in other cultures such changes are not seen with advancing age (Page and Sidd, 1972).

Jackson *et al.* (1976) found high blood pressures in healthy old people. This seems to indicate a confusion between asymptomatic and healthy. The large-scale follow-up studies, particularly the Framingham study, have firmly linked hypertension with cerebrovascular morbidity and mortality. So the concept of benign hypertension is no longer tenable. The serious prognostic significance for patients between 65 and 74 years of age, whose systolic pressure is greater than 180 mm Hg and diastolic blood pressure greater than 110 mm Hg, has been well described by Miall and Chinn (1974). The increased mortality with increasing blood pressure is probably as great for men as women (Chrysant *et al.*, 1976). Hypertensives with such a level of blood pressure have a four times greater risk of cardiovascular morbidity and mortality than those of the same age whose systolic blood pressure is less than 130 mm Hg. Hypertension is a potent cause of congestive cardiac failure. Kannel *et al.* (1972) showed from the Framingham study that 75% of patients with congestive cardiac failure were hypertensive and that this group exhibited a mortality seven times that of the general population. In terms of suffering and human misery the cost to the community from strokes, coronary artery disease, and congestive cardiac failure resulting from untreated hypertension is huge.

The *Lancet* editorial on hypertension in the elderly (Editorial, 1977) commented that 'In middle-aged men, the risks of stroke, dissecting aneurysm and cardiac failure, all common in the elderly, are substantially diminished by therapy so that it would be surprising if this were not at least partly true in later decades.' This is likely to be so, but it is also possible that the benefits in the elderly may be less and the risks greater. To decide this, a controlled clinical trial is required. The results of such a trial by the European Working Party on Hypertension in the Elderly are eagerly awaited. At present the best information on the effect of treatment in the aged is that of the Veterans Administration Co-operative Study Group on Antihypertensive Agents (1972). They showed that treatment for hypertension reduced the incidence of cerebrovascular accident from 23% to 8%, and of congestive cardiac failure from 21% to 0%.

The main argument put forward for not treating hypertension in the elderly is that by reducing blood pressure organ perfusion may be reduced with disastrous consequences. It does appear that, because of the arteriosclerotic vascular disease associated with age, there will in the elderly be a greater degree of irreversibility than in younger patients (Dunstan, 1974). There is, however, no evidence to show that the elderly are unable to maintain perfusion when the blood pressure is reduced in a careful manner. Cerebral autoregulation is disturbed in hypertensives of all ages and readjustment towards normal occurs with therapy despite the age of the patient (Strandgaard, 1976). Cerebral blood flow may in fact increase with therapy (Meyer *et al.*, 1968). Similar circulatory improvement with decreased vascular resistance has been shown in the kidneys (Dunstan, 1974; Koch-Weser, 1974). Whilst foolish therapy can have the disastrous consequences reported by Jackson *et al.* (1976), there is good evidence that the careful treatment of hypertension in the elderly can be achieved safely and reduce the risk of associated morbidity and mortality (Dyer *et al.*, 1977).

In the elderly the systolic pressure tends to rise more than the diastolic pressure (O'Rourke, 1970). O'Rourke explained this finding on the basis of an increased peripheral resistance leading to an elevation of the mean pressure. This results in an elevation of both systolic and diastolic pressure if the arterial distensibility is unaltered. However, arterial distensibility is often reduced in the elderly due to atherosclerosis. Then the systolic pressure increases more than the diastolic pressure, which may actually show a slight decrease. This greater elevation of systolic pressure which occurs with age has long been thought to be a relatively innocuous finding. This is not the case. In many instances the complications of hypertension (such as thrombotic stroke or LVH) have been shown to correlate more strongly with high systolic pressure than high diastolic pressure (Kannel *et al.*, 1972).

On the available evidence it would seem reasonable to treat an old person with a blood pressure above 180/105 and to aim for a standing diastolic pressure of 100 mm Hg during treatment. It is also important to treat obesity since this impairs the efficacy of therapy (Reisin *et al.*, 1978).

DRUG REGIMENS

Diuretics

Diuretics are effective in hypertension by reducing external cardiac work and left ventricular wall tension by decreasing arterial pressure. In hypertension the most useful diuretics are medium- and long-acting agents, e.g. thiazides, chlorthalidone, clorexolone, mefruside, and bumetanide (Davies and Wilson, 1975). In elderly patients who are not obese, the initial line of therapy would be a small dose of an oral thiazide, e.g. bendrofluazide 5 mg daily or hydrochlorothiazide 50–100 mg daily. It is essential to warn the patient that a diuresis will ensue. This is particularly true if the patient is in any way immobile or has any degree of incontinence—a patient totally demoralized by incontinence is unlikely to co-operate with therapy. The thiazides are relatively cheap but their great disadvantage is their impairment of carbohydrate metabolism (Editorial, 1978a). This is found to occur in 20% of patients taking the drug for more than 3 years. Some degree of hypokalaemia seems almost inevitable (Wilkinson *et al.*, 1975). This occurs early in treatment (Leemhuis and Struyvenberg, 1973; Morgan and Davidson, 1980). The controversy surrounding hypokalaemia and the use of potassium supplements or potassium-conserving drugs will be considered later in this chapter. The thiazide group of diuretics also enhances the action of other antihypertensive agents (Lindeman *et al.*, 1963; Beem and Mayer, 1958; Onesti and Moyer, 1967; Wilkins, 1959).

Frusemide can occasionally be helpful in patients where fluid retention is very marked or those verging on renal failure. In the main its rapid action is not suited to the elderly patient. Ethacrynic acid has no place in the routine management of hypertension in the elderly.

At present there is considerable controversy surrounding the whole question of potassium replacement during diuretic therapy. Williamson (1978) estimated that some 30% of the elderly population are receiving regular diuretic therapy. It would also seem that the elderly are slightly more prone to hypokalaemia than younger patients (Ibrahim *et al.*, 1978; Dall and Gardiner, 1971). This may partly be explained by poor diet: most elderly people have a potassium intake below 50 mmol/day (Macleod *et al.*, 1975). Decreased muscle bulk and reduced gastrointestinal absorption may also play a part. Other drugs such as carbenoxalone, licorice derivatives, and steroids also increase potassium loss.

Current evidence suggests that little change occurs in intracellular potassium until the plasma concentration drops below 3.0 mmol/l (Morgan, 1975). The acid–base state also influences serum potassium. The harmful effects of hypokalaemia are most probably dependent on the ratio between intracellular and extracellular potassium.

Potassium supplements can be most unpalatable. Patient compliance for Slow K tablets is among the worst of any tablets prescribed for geriatric patients (Macdonald *et al.*, 1977; Brooks *et al.*, 1971). These tablets can be difficult to swallow and cause considerable problems with oesophageal reflux. The effervescent preparations are also not well liked by the elderly (Editorial, 1978a). To have a useful effect, potassium must be given in a dose of at least 24 mmol/day. The commonly used doses have only a small effect on serum potassium in patients taking diuretics (Ramsay *et al.*, 1977; Schwartz and Schwartz, 1974). The supplements have no effect on the total body potassium, as the increased intake is balanced by an increased urinary excretion of potassium (Schwartz and Schwartz, 1974; Davidson *et al.*, 1978; Down *et al.*, 1972). The combined diuretic–potassium preparations are an irrational and expensive approach to the problem. The amount of diuretic in these preparations is usually not sufficient to produce hypokalaemia, and the accompanying dose of potassium (7–8 mmol) would not prevent or correct hypo-kalaemia.

It is the personal preference of the authors to prescribe a potassium-sparing diuretic where hypokalaemia is a problem. Where potassium depletion is due to diuretics, these drugs (amiloride, triamterene, and spironolactone) reduce urinary potassium loss and can increase total body potassium. They do not influence the total body potassium deficit which occurs in congestive cardiac failure (Davidson *et al.*, 1978). These drugs must never be given with potassium supplements, as there is a very real risk of fatal hyperkalaemia (Greenblatt and Koch-Weser, 1973). Several combined preparations have been marketed containing a potas-sium-sparing diuretic and a thiazide diuretic (e.g. amiloride and hydro-chlorothiazide). There is, however, evidence to suggest that the com-bined preparations are less effective than the separate preparations (Macleod *et al.*, 1975; Antcliff *et al.*, 1972; Hansen and Bender, 1967). The combined preparations also have higher doses of the thiazide diure-tic than one would initially use in the elderly. They also seem to aggra-vate carbohydrate intolerance more (Waal-Manning and Simpson, 1977). Greenblatt and Koch-Weser (1973) reported considerable prob-lems with spironolactone in the elderly, especially where the blood urea was elevated. Gynaecomastia can also be particularly troublesome in men. When triamterene was used in the elderly there was a significant incidence of nausea (Macdonald *et al.*, 1977). The authors therefore nor-mally use amiloride.

Other simple remedies need also be considered. These can play a sig-nificant role in obviating the need for potassium supplements. It should be remembered that the antihypertensive effect of thiazide diuretics is nearly maximal at very low doses, e.g. 5 mg bendrofluazide and 25 mg chlorthalidone (Bengtsson *et al.*, 1975). Little hypokalaemia is likely at these modest doses and very little thereapeutic benefit is gained by substantially increasing them. A modest reduction in daily salt intake (to 70–80 mmol/day) can greatly influence the potassium loss by reducing the quantity of diuretic required and because distal renal tubule excretion of potassium depends on the amount of sodium delivered here (Whight *et al.*, 1974). Such a modest reduction of salt intake can be achieved by avoiding salty foods and by not adding salt to food at the table. Where diuretics are being used for the treatment of cardiac failure, the loop diuretics produce less potassium loss than the equipotent dose of a thiazide diuretic.

It is also important to remember that many elderly people have mild ankle oedema totally unrelated to congestive cardiac failure. Since this is due to immobility and poor venous tone, diuretics are not appropriate.

Beta-blockers

There is some evidence to suggest that with age the pharmacology of the autonomic nervous system changes. This evidence is conflicting (de Champlain and Cousineau, 1977; Lake *et al.*, 1977; Sever *et al.*, 1977). In *in vitro* studies Shocken and Roth (1977) showed an age-related decline in the number of β-adrenoreceptors in the membrane fraction of lymphocytes. The remaining sites did not show any functional alteration. In clinical studies in elderly subjects the response of the heart rate to propranolol has been shown to be less (Conway *et al.*, 1971). More recent studies, using the dose–response curve to isoprenaline before and after the administration of propranolol, have enabled an affinity constant for propranolol binding to β-adrenoreceptors to be developed (McDevitt *et al.*, 1976). This affinity constant has been shown to correlate inversely with age (Vestal *et al.*, 1978).

There are also age-related changes in the pharmacokinetics of β-blockers. Castleden *et al.* (1975) found that after a 40 mg dose of propranolol peak blood levels were four times higher in the elderly than in the young. Half-life was also substantially longer. Alterations in hepatic clearance and metabolism were believed to account for this. The decline in renal function with age is thought to be the reason for the delay in the excretion of practolol (Castleden *et al.*, 1975).

However, despite these changes, this group of drugs causes fewer problems in the elderly than methyldopa. If the initial approach to the treatment of hypertension with a modest dose of diuretic has not been successful, and there is no heart block or congestive cardiac failure, then a cardioselective β-adrenoreceptor blocking agent would be the next choice. Atenolol in particular seems well tolerated in the elderly (Editorial, 1978b). It has the great advantage of once-daily oral administration. The usual starting dose is 50 mg once daily, with slow increments, if necessary, to a maximum of 200 mg daily. Side-effects to β-blockers are shown in Table 4.1.

Table 4.1   Side-effects and contraindications to the use of β-blockers

Contraindications	
Bronchospasm	Check for history of asthma/wheezing
Cardiac failure	
Impaired atrioventricular conduction	
Raynaud's phenomenon	Mostly with non-selective β-blockers
Side-effects	
Muscle cramps	Propranolol, pindalol
CNS upset	Propranolol, pindalol
Glucose intolerance	Non-selective β-blockers
Increased plasma triglycerides	
May cause/aggravate renal insufficiency	
Gastrointestinal upset	
Ileus	Oxprenolol
Impotence	
Peyronie's syndrome	
Weight gain	

Adrenergic neurone blockers

Guanethidine, bethanidine, and debrisoquine are not widely used in the elderly. They tend to cause severe postural hypotension, and have largely been superseded by less dangerous drugs.

Rauwolfia

Rauwolfia derivatives have been largely superseded in the United Kingdom. Their potential to cause severe depression and even suicide has been well documented. These effects are more common in the elderly (Lindeman *et al.*, 1963). However, there are still individual elderly patients whose hypertension has been controlled by rauwolfia for many years. If they have had no side-effects, it would seem reasonable to continue the drug in these patients.

104

CNS α-adrenoreceptor stimulants

Methlydopa

This drug interferes with chemical transmission at the post-ganglionic
nerve endings, producing a false and less potent neurotransmitter (α-
methyl noradrenaline) which blocks the adrengeric receptor sites resulting in a decrease in peripheral arteriolar resistance (Trinker, 1971). It
also diminishes central nervous sympathetic outflow by stimulating α-
adrenoreceptors (Page *et al.*, 1977). The absorption of an oral dose varies
from 8 to 62% (Kwan *et al.*, 1976). It can be an extremely useful drug
in younger subjects, but in the elderly side-effects are common and serious (see Table 4.2). It is particularly liable to cause drowsiness and frank
psychiatric disturbance in the elderly (Dollery and Harington, 1962).
Methyldopa should probably be reserved for cases where thiazide diuretics have been inadequate and β-blockers are contraindicated. Where
methyldopa is used, a small starting dose of 125 mg b.d., gradually
increasing to 250 mg t.d.s. is recommended. Because of the very real risk
of postural hypotension it is imperative that the blood pressure should
always be estimated both lying and standing.

Table 4.2   Side-effects of methyldopa

Side-effect	Action	Reference
Drowsiness	May need to stop	Macdonald *et al.*, 1977
Depression	Stop drug	Macdonald *et al.*, 1977
Dreams	Stop drug	Macdonald *et al.*, 1977
Haemolytic anaemia	Stop drug	Worlledge, 1969
Drug fever	Stop drug	Alarcon-Segovia, 1976
Liver damage	Stop drug	Rodman *et al.*, 1976
Fluid retension	Diuretic	
Lactation	Stop drug	
Reduced libido	Stop drug	Bauer *et al.*, 1973
Postural hypotension	Stop drug	Caird *et al.*, 1973
Myocarditis	Stop drug	Mullick and McAllister, 1977
Nasal congestion	Stop drug	Committee on the Safety of Medicines (personal communication)
Retroperitoneal fibrosis	Stop drug	Committee on the Safety of Medicines (personal communication)
Pulmonary reactions	Stop drug	Cole, 1977
SLE syndrome	Stop drug	Alarcon-Segovia, 1976

Clonidine

This drug stimulates the α-adrenoreceptors in the vasomotor centres, diminishing the sympathetic outflow. Cardiac output decreases and peripheral resistance is lowered. Postural hypotension is not troublesome in the young, but it can be a real problem in the elderly (Lund-Johansen, 1976). Drowsiness is also a major disadvantage in the elderly. It can be so severe as to render the patient incapable of performing the activities of everyday living (Macdougall *et al.*, 1970). Any sudden cessation of the drug can lead to severe rebound hypertension (Goldberg *et al.*, 1977). For these reasons the drug appears unsuited to the elderly.

OTHER DRUGS

Hydralazine has been little studied in the aged. Its increasing role in younger age groups and personal experience suggest that low doses may have a limited but useful role where thiazide plus β-blocker are inadequate. Side-effects are common (see Table 4.4) but are less frequent and less severe when starting on low doses and increasing dosage slowly.

Minoxidil, a potent vasodilator, has not been studied in the elderly and should probably only be considered in very refractory hypertension.

Table 4.3 shows suggested therapy schedules.

The available drugs and their side-effects are detailed in Table 4.4.

The treatment of hypertension after stroke is an area of considerable controversy. Whilst it does seem that there is some positive advantage in treating young patients following a stroke, the evidence about the effect

Table 4.3   Suggested approach to therapy of hypertension in the elderly

---

(A) Small dose of oral thiazide, e.g. 5 mg bendrofluazide
                          50–100 mg hydroclorothiazide
   Add small dose of potassium-sparing diuretic if hypokalaemia, e.g. amiloride 5 mg
   Other measures:
     Do not add salt to food once cooked
     Reduce weight if obese

(B) If therapy with thiazides not sufficient, use:
     (i) β-blocker if no cardiac failure
          Atenolol 50 mg daily in ONE dose (maximum 200 mg)
     (ii) If contraindications to β-blocker
          Methyldopa 125 mg b.d. (to max. 250 mg b.d. or t.d.s.)

Table 4.4   Side-effects of antihypertensive drugs

Thiazide diuretics
    Hypokalaemia
    Hyperuricaemia
    Impaired glucose tolerance
    Raised plasma triglycerides
    Skin rash—can precede a necrotizing vasculitis
    Peripheral ischaemia

Methyldopa—see Table 4.3

β-Blockers—see Table 4.2

Hydralazine
    Drug-induced lupus (mainly with >200 mg daily)
    Headache
    Nausea
    Nasal congestion
    Conjunctivitis
    Peripheral neuropathy

Prazosin
    First-dose phenomenon
    May precipitate angina
    Fluid retention
    Postural hypotension

Clonidine
    Postural hypotension
    Rebound hypertension

Minoxidil
    Reflex tachycardia
    Fluid retention
    Pericardial effusion
    Hirsutism

in the elderly is conflicting and indeed some reports indicate that it can be positively harmful (Carter, 1970; Adams, 1965; Merrett and Adams, 1965).

Digoxin

Probably more has been written about the use of digoxin in the elderly than almost any other topic in geriatric medicine. Yet despite the plethora of views, anecdotes, reports, etc., the main questions of how much and for how long still remain controversial. For many years digoxin has been considered to be the mainstay in the treatment of congestive cardiac failure. This view is now being challenged, with diuretics being promoted as the drug of choice in mild to moderate cardiac failure, with possibly the addition of a vasodilator where severe congestive cardiac failure exists (Lemberg, 1978).

Because of the narrow therapeutic margin of digoxin, any change in drug handling can have serious and potentially disastrous consequences for the patient. Unfortunately, the elderly bear the brunt of these toxic reactions; 5% of the elderly are taking digoxin and toxicity is common both at home and in hospital. The Glasgow Drug Surveillance Programme (1973–76) found that some 20% of patients receiving digoxin developed toxicity, the majority of them being over 65 years of age. Whiting *et al.* (1978) studied the use of digoxin in a group of 42 elderly patients and found that only one-third of them were receiving an ideal dose.

The main actions of digoxin are listed in Table 4.5. The available digitalis preparations are listed in Table 4.6. In the United Kingdom digoxin is used almost exclusively.

The pharmacokinetics of digoxin have been studied in detail in young healthy adult volunteers (Sumner *et al.*, 1976). Unfortunately, such detailed documentation in the elderly is still lacking. The effect of impaired renal function on the excretion of digoxin has been studied (Bloom and Nelp, 1966; Halkin *et al.*, 1975). Overall clearance of digoxin depends on the glomerular filtration rate and correlates well with creatinine clearance. In congestive cardiac failure, digoxin clearance may be reduced more than the renal function would indicate (Benowitz

Table 4.5   Actions of digoxin

Increases force of myocardial contraction
Increases refractory period of the A–V node
Increases refractory period of the Purkinje fibres
Inhibits Na^+ and K^+ transport at cell level
Increased excitability of the ventricle
Automaticity of subsidiary pacemakers enhanced

Table 4.6   Digitalis preparations

Ouabain—unreliable absorption
Deslanoside
Digoxin—most commonly used preparation
Digitoxin
Digitalis leaf—obsolete

and Meister, 1976). In these instances urea clearance seems a better marker (Halkin *et al.*, 1975). However, there are extrarenal routes of digoxin excretion—particularly biliary and gut excretion. These routes become increasingly important as renal function declines, either through age or disease. There is some evidence that with age and declining renal function the apparent volume of distribution of digoxin decreases (Jusko *et al.*, 1974; Aronson and Grahame-Smith, 1977; Caird and Kennedy, 1977). The reduction in lean body mass may be a factor in this change. Digoxin absorption appears to be unaltered in the aged. Digoxin has a very low degree of protein binding and a high volume of distribution, so age-related changes in protein binding (Hayes *et al.*, 1975; Wallace *et al.*, 1976) are unlikely to exert any serious influence on digoxin handling.

The main parameter of digoxin handling used to determine dosage is the digoxin clearance. The daily dose of digoxin should ideally replace the amount excreted via the kidneys and the extrarenal routes. The renal clearance corresponds to the creatinine clearance. Renal excretion is mainly as unchanged glycoside (Steiness, 1974), but tubular reabsorption (Doherty *et al.*, 1969) and tubular secretion (Marcus, 1972; Steiness, 1974; Whiting *et al.*, 1977) also occur. Extrarenal clearance declines with age, but the exact nature of the decline does not relate well to any parameter of hepatic or alimentary function (Roberts and Caird, 1976). Several attempts have been made to make mathematical models for digoxin dosage, either by computer studies or prediction nonograms (Kampmann *et al.*, 1974). Jelliffe *et al.* (1972) have shown that by using such methods toxicity reactions to digoxin and other cardiac glycosides could be reduced by 23%.

Much myth surrounds 'digitalization' schedules. In practice it is doubtful if large loading doses are necessary as there is a linear dose-contractile response (Lee *et al.*, 1972). The therapeutic range for digoxin is 1–2 ng/ml. Taylor *et al.* (1974) suggested that 0.25 mg/day without a loading dose was effective in the elderly, but even this can be toxic if there is a degree of renal impairment. Caird (1974) suggested that unless there was some urgency the calculated maintenance dose was sufficient and that a loading dose was unnecessary.

Because of the long half-life of digoxin there is no rational basis for the practice of administering digoxin in divided doses. Indeed, where patients are mentally frail this practice can be harmful as it increases the likelihood of confusion leading to overdosage. Complicated dosage schedules such as 'take on alternate days' or 'take for five days then omit two' are also best avoided. Since the introduction of the smaller dose tablets of digoxin it should now be possible to provide a sensible once-daily dose schedule for nearly all patients.

The regular use of plasma digoxin levels will not always exclude toxicity, as patients can experience toxicity within the normal 'therapeutic' range. They must never be relied upon to the exclusion of the clinical findings. If any doubt remains that a patient's symptoms could be due to digoxin toxicity then the only sensible course is to stop the drug and observe the patient.

Several authors have assessed factors influencing the bioavailability of digoxin. Gerson *et al.* (1980) studied the influence of gastrointestinal disease on digoxin absorption. Severe jejunal disease decreased the absorption but ileal disease and steatorrhoea had remarkably little effect. Digoxin absorption is unchanged by age *per se*. Digoxin absorption can also

Table 4.7   Drugs which influence the response to digoxin

Method of interference	Drug	Points
Decreased absorption	Antacids	Slow-dissolving digoxin only
Decreased absorption	Antidiarrhoeals	
Decreased absorption	Cholestyramine	Must give 8 h apart
Decreased absorption	Colestipol	Must give 8 h apart
Decreased absorption	Neomycin	Digoxin toxicity possible on stopping
Decreased absorption	PAS	
Decreased absorption	Phenytoin	
Decreased absorption	Sulphasalazine	
Increased absorption	Anticholinergics	Slow-dissolving digoxin only
Altered enterohepatic circulation	Colestipol	
Reduced renal excretion	Spironolactone Quinidine	
Induced hepatic metabolism	Phenytoin	Digitoxin only
	Phenylbutazone	Digitoxin only
	Rifampicin	Digitoxin only
	Phenobarbitone	
Increased tissue response	Calcium Diuretics Carbenoxolone Amphoteracin B	Via electrolyte upset
	Suxamethonium	
	Sympathomimetics	

be influenced by other drugs such as antacids and antidiarrhoeals (Binnion and McDermott, 1972). Other drugs can also influence metabolism by inducing hepatic metabolism (only important for digitoxin) or by reducing renal excretion. Tissue response to digoxin may be increased by electrolyte changes: hypokalaemia caused by diuretics, carbenoxolone, or amphoteracin B; hypercalcaemia caused by calcium salts; or hypomagnesaemia caused by diuretics.

The clinical manifestations of digoxin toxicity in the elderly can be quite different from those seen in the younger age group (Dall, 1965). Frequently confusion and frank psychiatric disturbance is the presentation rather than the more classical nausea, vomiting, and bradycardia. Visual upset is also commoner in the elderly. Digoxin toxicity can also cause virtually every known cardiac arrhythmia. In the elderly there are two particular situations which suggest toxicity: the worsening of congestive cardiac failure with a rising pulse rate and the conversion of atrial fibrillation into a regular rhythm at about 100 beats per minute (regular nodal rhythm is a common toxic arrhythmia). Side-effects are detailed in Table 4.8.

It is essential that any elderly patient receiving digoxin should be regularly monitored for developing hypokalaemia as this aggravates the development of toxicity. Dehydration must also be clinically evaluated. As mentioned above, hypercalcaemia and hypomagnesaemia are less common electrolyte causes of toxicity.

That digoxin can be extremely beneficial is without doubt. But it is equally true that it can also be extremely dangerous and cause much unwanted suffering. It is commonly prescribed in the elderly and there is good evidence that this is often without clinical justification (Landahl *et al.*, 1977).

Many cases of congestive cardiac failure in the elderly respond well to diuretics alone (Hull and MacKintosh, 1977). Where there was a clinical indication for the use of digoxin, this must be regularly reviewed. Dall (1970) and Johnston and McDevitt (1979) showed that a substantial number of patients could have digoxin discontinued with no detrimental effect whatsoever. Even where the initial reason for prescribing digoxin was sound, it is still possible to withdraw it safely where there is no evidence of heart failure and the patient is in sinus rhythm (Liverpool Therapeutics Group, 1978).

Thus digoxin is a drug to be used with caution and avoided if at all possible in the elderly. The main indications for its use in this age group are the acute treatment of congestive cardiac failure and left ventricular failure, and the control of ventricular rate in recurrent or continuous atrial arrythmias, especially atrial fibrillation.

Table 4.8   Side-effects of cardiac glycosides

Fatigue
Visual haziness and alterations in colour perception
Muscle weakness
Nausea and anorexia
Psychiatric symptoms or frank psychiatric upset
Abdominal pain
Dizziness
Headache
Retrosternal pain
Cardiac arrhythmias
   heart block
   ventricular ectopics
   bradycardia

TREATMENT OF CARDIAC FAILURE

In congestive cardiac failure, treatment should begin with diuretics. Digoxin may also be required in more severe cases, especially if atrial fibrillation is present. Long-term digoxin should be avoided if possible. There is growing interest in the use of vasodilators in cardiac failure. Most studies to date have been on younger patients in specialized units, but useful conclusions of more general applicability are beginning to emerge.

The role of vasodilators in chronic congestive cardiac failure is still uncertain (Editorial, 1978b). Hydralazine (25–100 mg 6–8 hourly) may well be the best oral agent: initial experience in geriatric patients has also been fairly promising. Where dyspnoea is a prominent symptom, indicating pulmonary congestion, long-acting nitrates such as isorbide (20–40 mg orally 4-hourly) may be added to hydralazine.

In acute left ventricular failure the standard treatment remains intravenous frusemide. Morphine still has a useful role. Recent work has shown that sublingual glyceryl trinitrate or nifedipine increase systemic venous pooling and reduce the 'pre-load' on the failing left ventricle. Their use is of proven benefit and will doubtless become more widespread: no specific experience in the elderly is currently available.

ANTIARRHYTHMIC DRUGS

The main antiarrhythmic drugs are listed in Table 4.9.

A number of cardiac arrhythmias are particularly common in the elderly and require a detailed mention: heart block, atrial fibrillation, premature ventricular contractions, and ventricular tachycardia.

Table 4.9 Main antiarrhythmic drugs

	Dose	Side-effects
Supraventricular		
Verapamil	1 mg/ml i.v. (max 10 mg)	Heart block
(Ca^{++} antagonist)	40–120 mg t.d.s. orally	Bradycardia
		Hypotension
		Care if digoxin, β-blockers
		Avoid in sick sinus A–V block
Digoxin	0.0625–0.25 mg daily	See Table 4.8
Ventricular/supraventricular		
Quinidine	Note half-life increases with age	Mainly used for cardio-version
	Test dose 200 mg first; 330–660 mg 8-hourly	
Disopyramide	Intravenous 2 mg/kg to max 150 mg	Hypotension VT
	300 mg oral load; then 100–150 mg 6-hourly	Dry mouth Blurred vision Constipation
Procainamide	Intravenous 100 mg bolus then 20 mg/ml to max 1 g in 1 h	Hypotension Heart block Contraindicated in myasthenia gravis Severe cardiac failure Renal failure
Lignocaine	75–100 mg i.v., then 10 mg/min for 20 min	
Others		
β-blockers	For inappropriate sinus tachycardia Chronic ventricular arrhythmias	
Phenytoin	Therapy of digitalis-induced arrhythmias	Hypotension Vertigo
	50–100 mg i.v. every 5 min to 1 g	Dysarthria Anaemia
	500 mg daily for 2 days then 400 mg daily	Lupus
Amiodarone	VF WPW syndrome 300–600 mg daily	Corneal microdeposits Photosensitivity
Bretylium	VF 1–2 mg/min i.v.	Hypotension

Heart block

Idiopathic heart block is common in patients over 65 years of age. The main underlying pathology seems to be fibrosis of the conducting system. A considerable number of patients require no active intervention. Active intervention is indicated firstly where the patient's exercise tolerance has been significantly reduced by diminished cardiac output. This usually occurs only when the heart rate is below 50 beats per minute. The second indication is the occurrence of Stokes-Adams attacks. Temporary cardiac stimulation can often be achieved by using isoprenaline or atropine. However, the only satisfactory treatment is the insertion of a pacemaker.

Atrial fibrillation

This is very common in the elderly. Many patients require no therapy. The usual feature necessitating treatment is the onset of cardiac failure. The treatment is based on digoxin and diuretics, the problems of which have already been considered. Whilst digoxin can be withdrawn without detriment in many cases in sinus rhythm, long-term digoxin treatment is inevitable if it is needed to control ventricular rate after the onset of atrial fibrillation.

Ventricular tachycardia and premature ventricular contractions

Most premature ventricular contractions are asymptomatic and require no active treatment. If, however, they are associated with ventricular tachycardia or occur after a myocardial infarction then therapy with lignocaine is indicated. In chronic ventricular arrhythmias quinidine, procainamide, and propranolol can be tried. The therapy needs to be suited to the individual patient (Opie, 1980). A sequence of drugs may need to be tried until the desired therapeutic effect is obtained.

Anti-anginal agents

The mainstay of the treatment of angina is glyceryl trinitrate. This drug is widely used with relatively little trouble. It seems to act in two ways (Kasparian *et al.*, 1975):

(1) It dilates non-ischaemic segments of cardiac collateral blood vessels resulting in a redistribution of blood towards ischaemic areas.

114

(2) It dilates the systematic veins and arterioles and, as a result, left ventricular pressure and hence myocardial oxygen consumption is reduced.

Glyceryl trinitrate is administered sublingually and is effective in 2–3 min with a duration of effect of 15–30 min. Its short duration of action is due to extensive first-pass hepatic metabolism. It can either be used to relieve the pain of angina, or can be taken prior to performing some activity which is likely to provoke an anginal attack (Aronow, 1972).

Elderly patients must be warned about the risk of postural hypotension and should avoid standing still after taking the tablets. If glyceryl trinitrate produces headache it is worth while trying isorbide dinitrate 5 mg sublingually or chewable. This drug often produces less headache but is more expensive.

If glyceryl trinitrate or one of the other nitrate preparations is not adequate then it may be necessary to use a β-adrenoreceptor blocking agent, provided there exists no contraindication to its use (see Table 4.1). Other drugs which may need to be considered are nifedipine and verapamil (calcium ion antagonists) and perhexilene. At present little is known about the possible problems caused by these drugs in the elderly.

It is also important to remember that reducing weight, stopping smoking, and avoiding the precipating activity may bring benefit.

POSTURAL HYPOTENSION

Postural hypotension (orthostatic hypotension) is common among the geriatric population (Rodstein and Zeman, 1957; Johnson et al., 1965; Caird et al., 1973). It can range from merely a mild dizziness to a disabling condition resulting in patients becoming bedfast. It is a common cause of falls, especially on rising from a chair or getting out of bed to go to the toilet. In all patients where postural hypotension is suspected, the blood pressure must be taken both lying and standing. It would be better still to make this a routine part of the examination of any elderly patient. If from the history there is a high probability of the patient having postural hypotension then it can be helpful to check the blood pressure in the sitting position to prevent an unnecessary fall (Caird and Judge, 1974). In some patients blood pressure drops steadily as they walk and this should be checked by getting the patient to walk a short distance and then measuring the blood pressure. Symptoms should only be attributed to postural hypotension if the systolic blood pressure drops to less than 100 mg Hg.

Postural hypotension is probably caused by the interaction of an autonomic disorder (Gross, 1970) and another factor such as ECG evidence of heart disease, varicose veins (Rodstein and Zeman, 1957), diffuse brain disease, hyponatraemia, urinary tract infection (Fine, 1969), anaemia, and perhaps most importantly drugs. Table 4.10 details the worst drugs in this respect. Johnson (1976) found that the autonomic deficit could be in any part of the reflex arc. Occasionally there is a definite neurogenic cause for the patient's postural hypotension (Johnson, 1976). The most common mechanisms are peripheral neuropathy or the Shy–Drager syndrome.

Where postural hypotension is due to current drug therapy then the causal drug should be removed. If a febrile illness or dehydration is contributing to the upset by volume depletion then this should be corrected. When more drastic measures are required it is best to start with the simplest. Elastic stockings can be beneficial if the patient has the dexterity to put them on. Elevating the head of the bed, teaching the patient to get out of bed in stages and how to get out of a chair correctly may also improve the situation.

It may be necessary to resort to drug therapy: fludrocortisone, indomethacin, or a combination of tyramine plus a monoamine oxidase inhibitor have been used. Fludrocortisone in doses of 0.1–0.3 mg/day should be tried first. The dose necessary to control the blood pressure unfortunately usually also produces oedema. Indomethacin may be beneficial. It increases the systemic vascular resistance by increasing the vasoconstriction caused by endogenous angiotensin II and noradrenaline from the remaining nerve endings. It also inhibits prostaglandin synthesis (Davies *et al.*, 1980). Indomethacin may also be given in conjunction with fludrocortisone, since both drugs increase the blood volume and

Table 4.10   Drugs causing hypotension

Antihypertensive agents
Morphine
Qunidine
Phenytoin
β-adrenoreceptor blocking agents (i.v.)
Diuretics (via hypovolaemia)
Glyceryl trinitrate
Phenothiazines—notably chloropromazine
Tricyclic antidepressants
Levodopa

116

increase the vascular smooth muscle sensitivity to noradrenaline. Indomethacin seems to be most helpful in autonomic failure and the Shy–
Drager syndrome (Spokes *et al.*, 1979).

The combination of tyramine and a monoamine oxidase inhibitor can
be very effective (Lewis *et al.*, 1972; Nanda *et al.*, 1975). Its major disadvantage is that it requires fanatical zeal in dose timing. Many geriatric
patients are quite incapable of this.

THE TREATMENT OF THROMBOEMBOLIC
DISEASE IN THE ELDERLY

There are several factors increasing the likelihood of a deep venous
thrombosis or a pulmonary embolus. These factors include: obesity,
immobility, varicose veins, diuretic therapy, and calf vein compression
due to bed rest or surgery. These risk factors are common in the elderly,
rendering them vulnerable to both deep venous thrombosis and pulmonary embolism.

As described in Chapter 2, there are substantially increased risks, particularly of bleeding, attached to the use of anticoagulants (both heparin
and the coumarins) in the elderly (Jicks *et al.*, 1968; Husted and
Andreasen, 1976). The alterations in the body's handling of anticoagulants with age are multifactorial (Shepherd *et al.*, 1977—see Chapter 2). One of the main factors seems to be the greater inhibition of clotting factor synthesis. Even where a reduced dose is given to an elderly
patient, the anticoagulant effect is often greater than in a younger
patient.

Anticoagulants are metabolized in the liver and excreted via the kidneys. Their use should be avoided where there is significant impairment
of either renal or hepatic function. There are also a number of clinically
important drug interactions: these are listed in Table 4.11. Other factors
affecting the response to anticoagulants are noted in Table 4.12.

Many pulmonary emboli are small and produce no symptoms. Some
cause collapse of lung tissue and associated haemodynamic upset, whilst
a goodly number are fatal. Most physicians would anticoagulate patients
who have suffered a pulmonary embolus. The therapy would be heparin
by infusion (40,000 units over 24 h) followed by oral anticoagulants. The
duration of the heparin infusion is again variable. In younger patients
oral anticoagulants would normally be continued for 3–6 months. If an
elderly patient is mentally frail or without good social support, it is sometimes necessary to prolong the hospital stay and discontinue anticoagulants at the time of discharge.

Table 4.11   Important drug reactions with anticoagulants

Drugs which increase anticoagulant action	*Drugs which decrease anticoagulant action*
Steroids	Barbiturates
Clofibrate	Chloral hydrate
Thyroxine	Dichloral phenazone
Glucagon	Glutethimide
Phenylbutazone	Rifampicin
Metronidazole	Griseofulvin
Quinidine	Chlorpropamide/tolbutamide
Salicylates	Phenytoin
Triclofos	
Antibiotics	
Allopurinol	
Cimetidine	
Dextropropoxyphene	
Cotrimoxazole	
INAH	
Chloramphenicol	
Amitryptiline	
Sulphonamides	

Table 4.12   Factors which alter responsiveness to anticoagulants

Increased response	*Decreased response*
Jaundice	Nephrotic syndrome
Malabsorption and starvation	Autosomal dominant hereditary
Hepatic disease	resistance
Congestive cardiac failure	
Hyperthyroidism	
Drugs—see Table 4.11	

The treatment of deep vein thrombosis (DVT) is more controversial. Not all forms of DVT carry the same risk of pulmonary embolus (Walker, 1972). Those affecting the iliofemoral segment carry a much higher risk of pulmonary embolus than those DVTs confined to the calf. Many physicians feel that these peripheral thromboses are unlikely to propagate proximally. However, the authors feel that there is still a substantial risk of embolization and consequently would anticoagulate such patients. Ultrasound and radiolabelled fibrinogen screening can be valuable in establishing the precise extent and site of the DVT. Phlebography is not without hazard in the elderly, and in the vast majority of old people it would not be justified.

In the main the treatment of a calf DVT is by anticoagulants, in the same manner as for pulmonary embolus. If the patient has a non-occlusive iliofemoral thrombosis then thrombectomy should be considered.

If superficial thrombophlebitis alone is present, then anticoagulants are not needed. A simple analgesic (not phenylbutazone) is sufficient. If, however, the thrombophlebitis continues to spread, then anticoagulants or venous ligation may need to be considered (Adar and Salzman, 1975).

It is important to try and prevent thromboses, especially following surgery, in the elderly. This is particularly true of the 'curse of elderly ladies'—fractured neck of femur. Low-dose heparin or dextran 70 are effective in preventing post-operative DVT (Roberts and Cotton, 1975; Smith *et al.*, 1978). Where the operation is not on the lower limb, calf stimulation or pneumatic leggings can be used. The only method shown to reduce the incidence of post-operative pulmonary emboli (especially after hip surgery) is oral anticoagulation (Morris and Mitchell, 1978). Table 4.13 shows suitable dosage schedules.

Aspirin

The role of aspirin is slowly being elucidated. It has not been shown to be effective in preventing DVTs following surgery (Morris and Mitchell, 1978). It does, however, exert a benefit in preventing transient ischaemic attacks and strokes in elderly men but not women. The dose is 1.2 g daily.

Dipyridamole

This drug enhances the effect of oral anticoagulants in preventing emboli from prosthetic heart valves, but its role in other thromboembolic problems is at present unclear.

Table 4.13   Schedule for prevention of operative deep venous thromboses

---

(a) Low-dose subcutaneous heparin
    5000 units 2 h before operation
    5000 units subcutaneously 12-hourly for 7 days

(b) Dextran 70
    500 ml during the operation, then
    500 ml dextran 70 every second day for 6 days
  (most useful where patient has a bleeding tendency)

(c) Oral anticoagulation

Other indications for anticoagulants, such as the prevention of embolism from prosthetic heart valves or in atrial fibrillation, are unchanged in the elderly.

REFERENCES AND BIBLIOGRAPHY

Adams, G. F. (1965) Prospects for patients with strokes: with special reference to the hypertensive hemiplegic. *Brit. Med. J.*, **2**, 253.

Adar, R. and Salzman, E. W. (1975) Treatment of thromboses of veins of the leg. *N. Engl. J. Med.*, **292**, 348.

Alarcon-Segovia, D. (1976) Drug induced antinuclear Abs and lupus syndrome. *Drugs*, **12**, 69.

Alderman, M. H. and Yano, K. (1976) How prevalence of hypertension varies as diagnostic criteria change. *Am. J. Med. Sci.*, **271**, 343–9.

Antcliff, A. C. *et al.* (1972) Amiloride hydrochloride combined with hydrochlorthiazide in the control of hypertension and plasma potassium levels. *Brit. J. Clin. Pract.*, **26**, 413–16.

Aronow, W. S. (1972) Medical treatment of angina pectoris (IV). Nitroglycerin. *Am. Heart J.*, **84**, 415.

Aronson, J. K. and Grahame-Smith, D. G. (1977) Monitoring digoxin therapy. *Brit. J. Clin. Pharmacol.*, **4**, 223–7.

Bauer, G. E. *et al.* (1973) Reversibility of side-effects of antihypertensive drugs. *Med. J. Aust.*, **1**, 930.

Beem, J. R. and Mayer, J. H. (1958) Antihypertensive therapy for the elderly patient. *Geriatrics*, **13**, 378.

Bengtsson, C. *et al.* (1975) The effect of different doses of chlorthalidone on blood pressure, serum potassium and water. *Brit. Med. J.*, **1**, 197–9.

Benowitz, N. L. and Meister, W. (1976) Pharmacokinetics in patients with cardiac failure. *Clin. Pharmacokinet.*, **1**, 389.

Binnion, P. F. and McDermott, M. (1972) Bioavailability of digoxin. *Lancet*, **2**, 592.

Bloom, P. M. and Nelp, W. B. (1966) Relationship of the excretion of tritiated digoxin to renal function. *Am. J. Med. Sci.*, **251**, 133–44.

Brooks, R. H. *et al.* (1971) Effectiveness of inpatient follow-up care. *New Engl. J. Med.*, **285**, 1509–14.

Caird, F. I. (1974) Metabolism of digoxin in relation to therapy in the elderly. *Gerontol. Clin.*, **16**, 68.

Caird, F. I. and Judge, T. G. (1974) *Assessment of the Elderly Patient.* Pitman Medical, London.

Caird, F. I. and Kennedy, R. D. (1977) Digitalis and digoxin detoxication in the elderly. *Age and Ageing*, **6**, 21–8.

Caird, F. I. *et al.* (1973) Effect of posture on blood pressure in the elderly. *Br. Heart J.*, **35**, 527–30.

Canadian Co-operative Study Group (1978) A randomised trial of aspirin and sulphapyrazone in threatened stroke. *New Engl. J. Med.*, **299**, 53.

Carey, R. M. *et al.* (1976) The Charlottesville Blood Pressure Study: value of repeated blood pressure measurements. *JAMA*, **236**, 847–51.

Carter, A. B. (1970) Hypertensive therapy in stroke survivors. *Lancet*, **1**, 485.

120

Castleden, C. M. *et al.* (1975) The effect of age on the plasma levels of practolol and propranolol. *Br. J. Clin. Pharmacol.*, **2**, 303–6.

Chrysant, S. G. *et al.* (1976) Why hypertension s so prevalent in the elderly and how to treat it. *Geriatrics*, **31**, 101–8.

Cole, P. (1977) Drug induced lung disease. *Drugs*, **13**, 422.

Conway, J. *et al.* (1971) Sympathetic nervous activity during exercise in relation to age. *Cardiovasc. Res.*, **5**, 577–81.

Dall, J. L. C. (1965) Digitalis intoxication in elderly patients. *Lancet*, **1**, 194.

Dall, J. L. C. (1970) Maintenance digoxin in the elderly. *Brit. Med. J.*, **2**, 705.

Dall, J. L. C. and Gardiner, H. S. (1971) The dietary intake of potassium by geriatric patients. *Gerontol. Clin.*, **13**, 119.

Davidson, C. *et al.* (1978) Effects of potassium supplements, spironalactone or amiloride on the potassium status of patients with heart failure. *Postgrad. Med. J.*, **54**, 405–9.

Davies, D. L. and Wilson, G. M. (1975) Diuretics: mechanism of action and clinical application. *Drugs*, **9**, 178.

Davies, I. B. *et al.* (1980) Indomethacin treatment of postural hypotension. *Brit. Med. J.*, **280**, 181.

De Champlain, J. and Cousineau, D. (1977) Lack of correlation between circulating catecholamines in hypertension. *N. Engl. J. Med.*, **297**, 672.

Doherty, J. E. *et al.* (1969) Localization of the extrarenal excretion of tritiated digoxin. *Am. J. Med. Sci.*, **258**, 181–9.

Dollery, C. T. and Harington, J. (1962) Methyldopa in hypertension. *Lancet*, **1**, 759.

Down, P. F. *et al.* (1972) Fate of potassium supplements in six outpatients receiving long term diuretics for oedematous disease. *Lancet*, **2**, 721–4.

Dunstan, H. P. (1974) Atherosclerosis complicating chronic hypertension. *Circulation*, **50**, 871–89.

Dyer, A. R. *et al.* (1977) Hypertension in the elderly. *Med. Clin. N. Am.*, **65**, 513.

Editorial (1977) Hypertension in the elderly. *Lancet*, **1**, 684–5.

Editorial (1978a) Diuretics in the elderly. *Brit. Med. J.*, **1**, 1092–3.

Editorial (1978b) Hypertension—which drug? *Brit. Med. J.*, **2**, 75.

Eisalo, A. *et al.* (1974) The effects of alprenolol in elderly patients with raised blood pressure. *Acta Med. Scand.* (Suppl.), **554**, 23–31.

Fields, W. S. *et al.* (1977) Controlled trial of aspirin in cerebral ischaemia. *Stroke*, **8**, 301.

Fine, W. (1969) Some common factors in the causation of hypertension. *Gerontol. Clin.*, **11**, 206–15.

Gerson, C. D. *et al.* (1980) The bioavailability of digoxin tablets in patients with gastro-intestinal dysfunction. *Am. J. Med.*, **69**, 43–9.

Glasgow Drug Surveillance Programme (1973–76) In J. Crooks and I. H. Stevenson (eds.), *Drugs in the Elderly*. Macmillan, London.

Goldberg, A. D. *et al.* (1977) Blood pressure and heart rate after withdrawal of antihypertensive drugs. *Brit. Med. J.*, **1**, 1243.

Greenblatt, D. J. and Koch-Weser, J. (1973) Adverse reactions to spironolactone. *JAMA*, **225**, 40–3.

Gross, M. (1970) The effect of posture on patients with cerebrovascular disease. *Q.J. Med.*, N.S., **39**, 485–91.

Halkin, H. *et al.* (1975) Determinants of the renal clearance of digoxin. *Clin. Pharmacol Ther.*, **17**, 385–94.

Hamilton, M. *et al.* (1954) The arterial pressure in the general population. *Clin. Sci. Molec. Med.*, **13**, 11.

Hansen, K. B. and Bender, A. D. (1967) Changes in serum potassium levels occurring in patients treated with triamterene and a triamterene–hydrochlorthiazide combination. *Clin. Pharmacol. Ther.*, **8**, 392–9.

Hayes, M. J. *et al.* (1975) Changes in drug metabolism with increasing age. *Brit. J. Clin. Pharmacol.*, **2**, 69–79.

Hull, S. M. and MacKintosh, A. (1977) The discontinuation of maintenance digoxin therapy in general practice. *Lancet*, **2**, 1054.

Husted, S. and Andreasen, F. (1976) Individual variation in long-term treatment with anticoagulants. *Acta Med. Scand.*, **200**, 379.

Ibrahim, I. K. *et al.* (1978) Are potassium supplements for the elderly necessary? *Age and Ageing*, **7**, 165–70.

Jackson, G. *et al.* (1976) Inappropriate antihypertensive therapy in the elderly. *Lancet*, **2**, 1317–18.

Jelliffe, R. W. *et al.* (1972) Reduction in digitalis toxicity by computer assisted glycoside dosage regimens. *Ann. Intern. Med.*, **77**, 891–907.

Jicks, H. *et al.* (1968) Efficacy and toxicity of heparin in relation to age and sex. *N. Engl. J. Med.*, **279**, 284.

Johnson, R. H. (1976) In F. I. Caird, J. L. C. Dall, and R. D. Kennedy (eds), *Cardiology in Old Age*. Plenum Press, New York and London.

Johnson, R. H. *et al.* (1965) The effect of posture on blood pressure in elderly patients. *Lancet*, **1**, 731–3.

Johnston, G. D. and McDevitt, D. G. (1979) Is maintenance digoxin necessary in patients in sinus rhythm? *Lancet*, **1**, 567.

Jusko, W. J. *et al.* (1974) Pharmacokinetic design of digoxin dosage regimens in relation to renal function. *J. Clin. Pharmacol.*, **14**, 525–35.

Kampmann, J. *et al.* (1974) Rapid evaluation of creatinine clearance. *Acta Med. Scand.*, **196**, 517–20.

Kannel, W. B. *et al.* (1972) The role of blood pressure in the development of C.C.F. *New Engl. J. Med.*, **287**, 781–7.

Kannel, W. B. and Gordon, T. (eds) (1974) *The Framingham Study: an epidemiological investigation of cardiovascular disease*. US Govt. Printing Office, Washington, DC.

Kasparian, H. *et al.* (1975) Comparative haemodynamic effects of placebo and oral isosorbide dinitrate in coronary artery disease. *Am. Heart J.*, **90**, 68.

Koch-Weser, J. (1974) Vasodilator drugs in the treatment of hypertension. *Arch. Intern. Med.*, **133**, 1017–23.

Kwan, K. C. *et al.* (1976) Pharmacokinetics of methyldopa in men. *J. Pharmacol. Ther.*, **198**, 264.

Lake, C. R. *et al.* (1977) Age adjusted plasma norepinephrine levels in normal and hypertensive subjects. *New Engl. J. Med.*, **296**, 208–9.

Landahl, S. *et al.* (1977) Digitalis therapy in a 70 year old population. *Acta Med. Scand.*, **202**, 437.

Lee, G. *et al.* (1972) Demonstration of linear dose–response of digitalis. *Chest*, **62**, 367.

122

Leemhuis, M. P. and Struyvenberg, A. (1973) Significance of hypokalaemia due to diuretics. *Neth. J. Med.*, **16**, 18–28.

Lemberg, L. (1978) Digitalis in congestive heart failure: fact or fancy. *Arch. Intern. Med.*, **138**, 737.

Lewis, R. K. *et al.* (1972) Therapy of idiopathic postural hypotension. *Arch. Intern. Med.*, **129**, 943–9.

Lindeman, R. D. *et al.* (1963) Effect of hydrochlorothiazide and reserpine on cerebral function in elderly hypertensive patients. *J. Am. Ger. Soc.*, **2**, 597–606.

Liverpool Therapeutics Group (1978) Use of digitalis in general practice. *Brit. Med. J.*, **2**, 673.

Lund-Johansen, P. (1976) *Haemodynamic Effects of Clonidine in Man in Regulation of Blood Pressure.* Grune Stratton, New York.

Lundborg, P. and Steen, B. (1976) Plasma levels and effect on heart rate and blood pressure of metoprolol after acute oral administration in 12 geriatric patients. *Acta Med. Scand.*, **200**, 397–402.

McDevitt, D. G. *et al.* (1976) Plasma binding and the affinity of propranolol for β-adrenoreceptors in man. *Clin. Pharmacol. Ther.*, **17**, 21–30.

Macdonald, E. T. *et al.* (1977) Methods of improving compliance after hospital discharge. *Brit. Med. J.*, **2**, 618.

Macdougall, A. I. *et al.* (1970) Treatment of hypertension with clonidine. *Brit. Med. J.*, **3**, 440.

Macfarlane, I. F. R. and Kennedy, R. D. (1973) Clinical experience with amiloride in the elderly. *Acta Cardiol.*, **28**, 365–74.

Macleod, C. C. *et al.* (1975) Nutrition of the elderly at home. III. Intake of minerals. *Age and Ageing*, **4**, 49–57.

Marcus, F. I. (1972) Metabolic factors in determining digitalis dosage in man. In Marks,   . and Weissler,   . (eds), *Basic Clinical Pharmacology of Digoxin.* Thomas, Springfield, Ill.

Master, A. M. (1952) *Normal Blood Pressure and Hypertension.* Lea & Febiger, Philadelphia.

Master, A. M. and Laser, R. P. (1961) Blood pressure elevation in the elderly. In A. N. Brest and J. A. H. Moyer (eds), *Recent Advances in Hypertension.* Lea & Febiger, Philadelphia.

Merrett, J. D. and Adams, G. F. (1965) Comparison of mortality rates in elderly hypertensive and normotensive hemiplegic patients. *Brit. Med. J.*, **2**, 802.

Meyer, J. S. *et al.* (1968) Cerebral blood flow after control of hypertension. *Neurology*, **18**, 772–81.

Miall, W. E. and Chinn, S. (1974) Screening for hypertension: some epidemiological observations. *Brit. Med. J.*, **3**, 595–600.

Morgan, D. B. and Davidson, R. (1980) Hypokalaemia and diuretics: an analysis of publications. *Brit. Med. J.*, **1**, 905.

Morris, G. K. and Mitchell, J. R. A. (1977) Preventing D.V.T. in elderly patients with hip fractures: studies of low dose heparin, dipyridamole, aspirin and flurbiprofen. *Brit. Med. J.*, **1**, 535.

Morris, G. K. and Mitchell, J. R. A. (1978) Prevention of death from D.V.T. in the elderly. *Am. Heart J.*, **95**, 139.

Mullick, F. G. and McAllister, H. A. (1977) Myocarditis associated with methyldopa. *JAMA*, **237**, 1699.

Nanda, R. N. *et al.* (1975) Treatment of neurogenic orthostatic postural hypotension with monamine oxidase inhibitors and tyramine. *Clin. Sci. Molec. Med.*, **49**, 13P.

Onesti, G. and Moyer, J. H. (1967) Hypertension in the past 60 years. *Geriatrics*, **22**, 192.

Opie, L. H. (1980) Which drug for which disease? *Lancet*, **1**, 1011–17.

O'Rourke, M. F. (1970) Arterial haemodynamics in hypertension. *Circ. Res.*, **26–27** (Suppl. 2), 123.

Page, L. B. *et al.* (1977) Drugs in the management of hypertension. II. *Am. Heart J.*, **92**, 144.

Page, L. B. and Sidd, J. J. (1972) Medical management of hypertension. *New Engl. J. Med.*, **287**, 960–7.

Ramsay, L. E. *et al.* (1977) Factors influencing serum potassium in treated hypertension. *Q.J. Med.*, **46**, 401–10.

Reisin, E. *et al.* (1978) Effect of weight loss without salt restriction in the reduction of blood pressure in overweight hypertensive patients. *New Engl. J. Med.*, **298**, 1.

Roberts, M. A. and Caird, F. I. (1976) Steady-state kinetics of digoxin in the elderly. *Age and Ageing*, **5**, 214–23.

Roberts, V. C. and Cotton, L. T. (1975) Low dose heparin and calf compression. *Brit. Med. J.*, **3**, 458.

Rodman, J. S. *et al.* (1976) Methyldopa hepatitis. *Am. J. Med.*, **60**, 941.

Rodstein, M. and Zeman, F. D. (1957) Postural blood pressure changes in the elderly. *J. Chron. Dis.*, **6**, 581–8.

Schwartz, A. B. and Schwartz, M. D. (1974) Dosage of potassium chloride elixir to correct thiazide-induced hypokalaemia. *JAMA*, **230**, 702–4.

Sever, P. S. *et al.* (1977) Plasma noradrenaline in essential hypertension. *Lancet*, **1**, 1078–81.

Shepherd, A. M. M. *et al.* (1977) Age as a determinant of sensitivity to renal function. *Brit. J. Clin. Pharmacol.*, **4**, 315.

Shocken, D. and Roth, G. (1977) Reduced beta-adrenergic receptor concentrations in ageing man. *Nature*, **267**, 856–8.

Smith, R. C. *et al.* (1978) Dextran and intermittent pneumatic compression in prevention of post-operative D.V.T. *Brit. Med. J.*, **1**, 952.

Society of Actuaries (1959) *Build and Blood Pressure Study.* Chicago.

Spokes, E. G. S. *et al.* (1979) Multiple system atrophy with autonomic failure: clinical, histological, and neurochemical observations on four cases. *J. Neurol. Sci.*, **45**, 59–82.

Steiness, E. (1974) Renal tubular secretion of digoxin. *Circulation*, **50**, 103–7.

Strandgaard, S. (1976) Autoregulation of cerebral blood flow in hypertensive patients. *Circulation*, **53**, 720–7.

Sumner, D. J. *et al.* (1976) Digoxin pharmacokinetics—multicompartmental analysis. *Br. J. Clin. Pharmacol.*, **3**, 221–9.

Taylor, B. B. *et al.* (1974) Digoxin studies in the elderly. *Age and Ageing*, **3**, 79–84.

Trinker, F. R. (1971) The significance of the relative potencies of N.A. and methyl N.A. for the mode of action of methyldopa. *J. Pharm. Pharmacol.*, **23**, 306.

124

United States National Centre for Health Statistics (1977) *Blood Pressure Levels of Persons 6–74 Years*. U.S. Govt. Printing Office. Series II, No. 203, Rockville, Maryland.

Vestal, R. E. *et al.* (1978) Reduced β-adrenoreceptor sensitivity in the elderly. *Clin. Res.*, **26**, 488A.

Veterans Administration Co-operative Study Group (1972) Effects of treatment on morbidity in hypertension (III). *Circulation*, **45**, 991–1004.

Waal-Manning, H. J. and Simpson, F. O. (1977) A fixed combination of amiloride hydrochloride and hydrochlorothiazide. In Magnami, . (ed.), *Diuresis, Kaliuresis and Hypertension*. Futura Publishing, New York.

Walker, M. G. (1972) The natural history of venous thromboembolism. *Br. J. Surg.*, **124**, 169.

Wallace, S. *et al.* (1976) Factors affecting drug binding in plasma of elderly patients. *Br. J. Clin. Pharmacol.*, **3**, 327–30.

Whight, C. *et al.* (1974) Diuretics, cardiac failure and potassium depletion: a rational approach. *Med. J. Aust.*, **2**, 831–3.

Whiting, B. *et al.* (1978) A computer assisted review of digoxin therapy in the elderly. *Br. Heart J.*, **40**, 8–13.

Wilkins, R. W. (1959) Drug therapy of hypertension in old age. *Postgrad. Med. J.*, **26**, 59.

Wilkinson, P. R. *et al.* (1975) Total body and serum potassium during prolonged thiazide therapy for essential hypertension. *Lancet*, **1**, 759.

Williamson, J. (1978) Prescribing problems in the elderly. *Practitioner*, **220**, 749–55.

Worlledge, S. M. (1969) Immune drug induced haemolytic anaemias. *Sem. Haematol.*, **6**, 181.

Chapter 5

Antibiotics and the aged

Antibiotics can be lifesaving. They are also among the most misused and abused drugs in medical practice. The cost of this abuse is great, both to the patient and the community. The patient pays with unnecessary mortality and morbidity due to drug reactions. The community pays in the cost of unnecessary prescriptions and also more importantly in the obsolescence of valuable drugs. A recently conducted survey (Moss *et al.*, 1981a) found that in hospital practice over a third of the courses of antibiotics prescribed were unjustified. It also found that as one got older the chances of being prescribed antibiotics rise sharply, as does the likelihood of this therapy being unwarranted. It is obvious that a far more careful approach is required if the use of these drugs is to be improved.

No difficulties of choice exist at the extremes of severe bacterial infection, when antibiotics can be lifesaving, and trivial infections in otherwise healthy patients, when antibiotics are not indicated. The middle ground is a much more difficult area. It is here that improved clinical techniques could produce the greatest benefits both in terms of health care and cost.

The signs of infection which one sees in the younger age group can in the elderly be very muted and easily missed. One of the commonest presentations of infection in the elderly is as a toxic confusional state. Even relatively trivial infections can produce this effect. It is also important to remember that the upper limit of normal for the total white cell count is lower than in young adults ($9000/mm^3$ as opposed to $10–11,000/mm^3$ in the younger patient). If this is not borne in mind, the leucocytosis of infection may be missed.

The bacteriological principles which would be applied to the treatment of infection in the young apply just as much to the elderly. These principles are summarized in Table 5.1.

It is not always possible to have a definite bacteriological diagnosis prior to the start of therapy. In these instances, before treatment is commenced the appropriate samples (sputum, urine, blood, CSF, etc.) should be obtained. Blood cultures can be very helpful in establishing the nature of the causative organism in the elderly. In younger age groups (12–49 years) only some 7% of blood cultures yield positive results. This contrasts with the fact that more than 50% of blood cultures will be positive in those over 60 years (Austrian, 1968). They are, however, worthless if the technique used to obtain them is not scrupulously aseptic. Where therapy has to be started prior to bacterial confirmation and sensitivity, it is essential that the choice of drug should be based on a sound knowledge of the prevalent organisms and their resistance patterns. This applies both to patients in the community and in hospital.

Elderly patients admitted to hospital are frequently diagnosed as having lower respiratory tract infections. Sadly, this diagnosis has been shown to be erroneous in a substantial number of cases (Moss *et al.*, 1981b). The most common error is the incorrect interpretation of chest X-ray findings (usually mistaking pulmonary oedema for infection). It is

Table 5.1   Principles of antibacterial therapy in the elderly

---

(1) *Clinical assessment*
  (a) Determine site of infection.
  (b) Severity of infection—use drugs only when needed.
  (c) Drug cultures and other diagnostic specimens taken prior to start of therapy.

(2) *Organism*
  (a) Identify organism.
  (b) Find drug sensitivity of organism.
  (c) Question strange results.

(3) *Nature of drug*
  (a) Best drug for particular site and organism.
  (b) Always use the least toxic of the available effective drugs.
  (c) Do you require more than one drug to prevent resistance, e.g. multiple drug therapy for pulmonary tuberculosis?
  (d) Risk of toxicity reactions with other drugs being administered.

(4) *Patient characteristics*
  (a) Age—smaller doses may be required to avoid toxicity, e.g. streptomycin.
  (b) Renal impairment—some drugs best avoided.
  (c) Hepatic disease.
  (d) Allergic response—avoid penicillins where previous allergic reaction.
  (e) Other diseases.

(5) *Choice of individual drug from the therapeutic class*
  (a) Most effectively absorbed.
  (b) Influence of protein binding on bacterial activity.
  (c) Route of administration.
  (d) Frequency of dose.
  (e) How common are side-effects?
  (f) Gravity of side-effects?
  (g) Cost of treatment.

---

vitally important that a thorough clinical examination be carried out prior to the commencement of antibacterial therapy. Matters would also be improved by a more thorough grounding in X-ray interpretation for all doctors dealing routinely with unreported emergency X-ray films.

A similarly large number of patients are treated for urinary tract infections in the absence of corroboration. It is extremely unlikely that symptoms are due to urinary tract infection in the absence of significant bacteriuria (>100,000 organisms/ml) (Asscher, 1977). Pyuria should be looked for in every case.

It is also preferable to use a bactericidal rather than a bacteriostatic antibiotic when treating infections in the elderly.

Four main factors govern the dosage of antibiotic required for an elderly patient:

(1) the elderly have a lower body weight than the young subjects in whom the normal dose is fixed;
(2) hepatic and renal function decline with age;
(3) the elderly are frequently on multiple-drug therapy, resulting in competition for binding sites;
(4) the renal function in healthy elderly patients is not necessarily the same as the sick elderly (Denham *et al.*, 1975).

Some studies have been carried out to elucidate changes in the handling of antibiotics with age. These changes are detailed in Table 5.2.

The main antibacterial drug categories are detailed in Table 5.3 and their clinical application is detailed in Table 5.4.

One very important aspect of antibacterial therapy in the elderly is the

Table 5.2   Studies on pharmacokinetics and pharmacodynamics of antibiotics in the elderly

Drug	Finding	Reference
Penicillin G	No alteration in absorption	Leikola and Vartia,
Procaine penicillin	Higher serum levels	1957
Dihydrostreptomycin	Higher serum levels due to	Vartia and Leikola,
Tetracycline	reduced excretion	1960
Propicillin	Decreased volume of distribution	Simon *et al.*, 1972
INAH	Apparently unchanged	Bender, 1968
Penicillin G	Increased half-life	Molholm-Hansen *et al.*, 1970
Amoxycillin	Increased half-life	Ball *et al.*, 1978

128

Table 5.3   The main antibacterial drug classes

(1) *Penicillins*
    (a) *Penicillinase-sensitive*
        Benzylpenicillin
        Procaine penicillin
        Benethamine penicillin
        Phenoxymethylpenicillin
    (b) *Penicillinase-resistant*
        Cloxacillin
        Flucloxacillin
        Methicillin sodium
    (c) *Broad-spectrum penicillins*
        Amoxycillin
        Ampicillin
        Ciclacillin
        Pivampicillin
        Talampicillin hydrochloride
    (d) *Penicillins effective against Pseudomonas infections*
        Carbenicillin
        Carfecillin sodium
        Mezlocillin sodium
        Ticarcillin sodium

(2) *Cephalosporins and cephamycin*
    Cefaclor
    Cefoxitin
    Cefuroxime
    Cephalexin
    Cephaloridine
    Cephalothin
    Cephamandole macate
    Cephazolin
    Cephradine

(3) *Tetracyclines*
    Tetracycline
    Chlortetracycline hydrochloride
    Clomocycline sodium
    Demeclocycline hydrochloride
    Doxycycline
    Lymecycline
    Methacycline hydrochloride
    Minocycline
    Oxytetracycline

(4) *Aminoglycosides*
    Gentamicin
    Amikacin sulphate
    Framycetin sulphate

Table 5.3   continued

Kanamycin
Neomycin sulphate
Tobramycin

(5) *Macrolides*
Erythromycin
Spiromycin
Clindamycin
Lincomycin

(6) *Others*
Chloramphenicol
Colistin
Sodium fusidate
Novobiocin
Polymyxin B
Cotrimoxazole
Sulphonamides

(7) *Antituberculous drugs*
Isoniazid
Rifampicin
Ethambutol
Streptomycin
PAS
Pyrazinamide
Capreomycin
Cycloserine
Ethionamide

(8) *Urinary antimicrobial drugs*
Nitrofurantoin
Cinoxacin
Nalidixic acid

---

greater risk of drug interaction due to polypharmacy. These reactions are of three main types (Kabins, 1972):

(1) displacement from serum protein carrier sites—e.g. sulphonamides, cotrimoxazole and nalidixic acid all compete for serum protein sites with warfarin.
(2) Interaction with liver enzymes—e.g. chloramphenicol, cotrimoxazole and sulphonamides diminish the activity of liver enzymes in dealing with anticoagulants. Griseofulvin, on the contrary, increases this activity. All broad-spectrum antibiotics inhibit the production of vitamin K in the gut. These drugs also decrease the liver

Table 5.4 Clinical applications of antibacterial drugs

Infection	Suggested therapy
Respiratory infections	
Acute bronchitis	Amoxycillin, 250 mg 8-hourly—may increase to 500 mg 8-hourly in severe infection Cotrimoxazole, 960 mg 12-hourly
Pneumonia	
no chest history	Amoxycillin, 500 mg 8-hourly
history of chest disease	Amoxycillin, 500 mg 8-hourly
Tuberculosis	Rifampicin, 450 mg daily (600 mg if >50 kg) Isoniazid, 300 mg daily Ethambutol*, 15 mg/kg
Gastrointestinal system infections	
Salmonellosis	Ampicillin, 0.25–1 g 6-hourly Cotrimoxazole, 960 mg 12-hourly
Biliary tract infection	Amoxycillin, 500 mg 8-hourly
Cardioavascular system infections	
Endocarditis	
Staph. aureus	Flucloxacillin, 500 mg 6-hourly
Strep. viridans	Benzylpenicillin and gentamicin†
Strep. faecalis	Benzylpenicillin and gentamicin, up to 24 g daily; 2–5 mg/kg 12-hourly
Central nervous system infections	
Meningitis	Benzylpenicillin, up to 24 g daily (chloramphenicol if *H. influenzae*)
Urogenital infections	
Acute pyelonephritis	Cotrimoxazole, 960 mg daily
Acute prostatitis	Cotrimoxazole, 960 mg daily
'UTI'	Ampicillin, 0.25–1 g daily
'Recurrent UTI'	Ampicillin, 0.25–1 g daily Cotrimoxazole, 960 mg daily

* *Ethambutol*: optic toxicity has not been found to be a problem in the elderly when dose used is 15 mg/kg (Doster *et al.*, 1973).

† *Gentamicin*: monitor by serum concentrations. The level 1 h after injection should not exceed 110 µg/ml and the pre-dose concentrations should not exceed 1 µg/ml.

    Where significant renal impairment the dosage interval should be prolonged:
    12 hourly if creatinine clearance in the range 30–70 ml/min
    24 hourly if creatinine clearance in the range 10–30 ml/min

Table 5.5   Antibiotics and renal impairment

Antibiotic	Nature of renal impairment	Toxic effect
Gentamicin	Impaired renal excretion	Ototoxicity
Streptomycin		Nephrotoxicity
Kanamycin		
Tobramycin		
Amikacin		
Neomycin		
Vancomycin		
Colistin	Decreased excretion	Neurotoxicity
Polymyxin		Nephrotoxicity
Cotrimoxazole	Hypersensitivity to sulphonamide	Nephrotoxic
Tetracyclines	Impaired excretion	Elevates blood urea
	Altered metabolism	Aggravates renal insufficiency (not doxycycline and minocycline)
Penicillins	Impaired excretion	Convulsions
	Accumulation of K^+ & Na^+ salts	Haemolytic anaemia
		High K^+ Na^+ levels
Carbenicillin	Impaired excretion	Bleeding, acidosis
		Hypernatraemia
Methicillin	Impaired excretion	Allergic interstitial nephritis
Cephalosporins	Impaired renal excretion	Nephrotoxicity
		Haemolytic anaemia
Chloramphenicol	Impaired renal excretion	Bone marrow toxicity from accumulated metabolites
Nitrofurantoin		Crystalluria
		Inadequate urine levels
		Neuropathy
		Pulmonary toxicity
Sulphonamides		Crystalluria
Nalidixic acid		Neurotoxicity

breakdown of oral hypoglycaemic agents, particularly tolbutamide.

(3) Competition for tubular excretion in the kidney—e.g. sulphonamides and septrin compete for the binding sites for tubular excretion with the sulphonylureas.

The absorption of many antibiotics (penicillins, sulphonamides, nitro-

132

furantoin, and tetracyclines) can be adversely affected by the concomitant administration of antacids, or being taken with food.

It is also very important to bear in mind that frusemide and potassium-losing diuretics can be nephrotoxic when administered with cephaloridine and cephalothin. The problems of using antibiotics in the presence of renal impairment are summarized in Table 5.5.

Sadly, antibiotics seem to be widely misused (Moss *et al.*, 1981 a, b, and c). The commonest mistakes are inadequate cover for the likely organism, inappropriate drug therapy, and unsuitable combinations of drugs. It is also true that these valuable drugs are being widely used where there is no real clinical indication to do so. This could be avoided if doctors were more scrupulous in their prescribing. A scoring system (Moss *et al.*, 1981b) based on various diagnostic features such as leucocytosis, temperature, clinical state, sputum/urine examination, other diseases such as diabetes, and concomitant therapy with drugs such as corticosteroids or immunosuppressives may help to improve their application.

Figure 5.1 provides a checklist for infections in the elderly.

REFERENCES AND BIBLIOGRAPHY

Asscher, A. W. (1977) Diseases of the urinary system: urinary tract infections. *Brit. Med. J.*, **1**, 1332–5.

Austrian, R. (1968) Current status of bacterial pneumonia with special reference to pneumococcal infections. *J. Clin. Pathol.* (suppl.), **21**, 93.

Ball, P. *et al.* (1978) Prolonged serum elimination half-life of amoxycillin in the elderly. *J. Antimicrob. Chemother.*, **4**, 385.

Bender, A. D. (1968) Effect of age on intestinal absorption: implications for drug absorption in the elderly. *J. Am. Geriat. Soc.*, **16**, 1331–9.

Denham, M. J. *et al.* (1975) Glomerular filtration in sick patients. *Age and Ageing*, **4**, 32.

Doster, B. *et al.* (1973) Ethambutol in the initial treatment of pulmonary tuberculosis. *Am. Rev. of Resp. Dis.*, **107**, 177.

Kabins, S. A. (1972) Interactions among antibiotics and other drugs. *JAMA*, **219**, 206.

Leikola, E. and Vartia, K. O. (1957) On penicillin levels in young and geriatric subjects. *J. Gerontol.*, **12**, 48–52.

Molholm-Hansen, J. M. *et al.* (1970) Renal excretion of drugs in the elderly. *Lancet*, **1**, 1170.

Moss, F. *et al.* (1981a) Survey of antibiotic prescribing in a district general hospital—(1) Patterns of use. *Lancet*, **2**, 349–52.

Moss, F. *et al.* (1981b) Survey of antibiotic prescribing in a district general hospital—(2) Lower respiratory tract infection. *Lancet*, **2**, 407–9.

Moss, F. *et al.* (1981c) Survey of antibiotic prescribing in a district general hospital—(3) Urinary tract infection. *Lancet*, **2**, 461–2.

Simon, C. *et al.* (1972) Zur Pharmakokinetik von Propicillin bei geriatrischen Patienten im Vergleich zu jungeren Erwachsenen. *Deutsch. Med. Wschr.*, **97**, 1999–2003.
Vartia, K. O. and Leikola, E. (1960) Serum levels of antibiotics in young and old subjects following administration of dihydrostreptomycin and tetracycline. *J. Gerontol.*, **12**, 48–52.

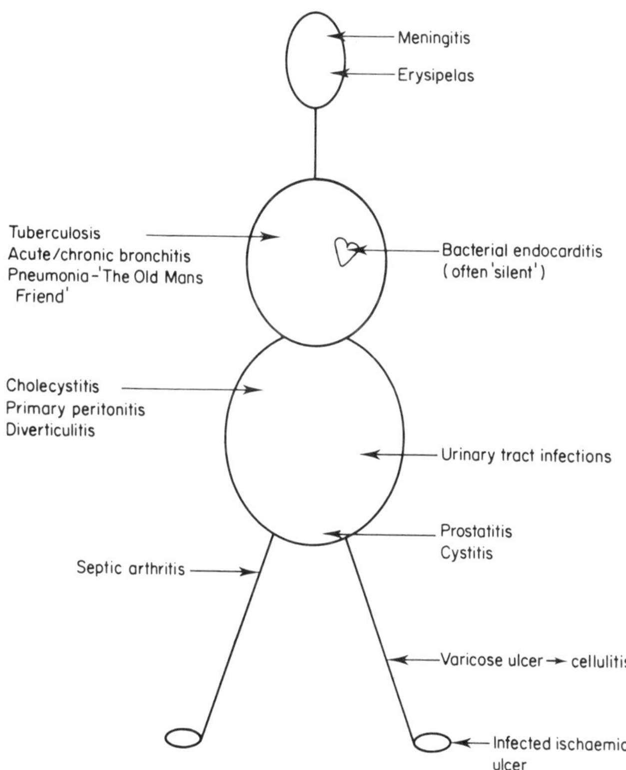

Fig. 5.1   Checklist of infections

Chapter 6

Metabolic and endocrine diseases

The main physiological effects of age on the endocrine system have been detailed in Chapter 1. The reader is also recommended two excellent review articles (Gregerman and Bierman, 1974; Andres and Tobin, 1977).

The most common metabolic disease in the elderly is diabetes. However, its diagnosis is not as straightforward as one might expect. The glucose tolerance changes with advancing years (Butterfield, 1964). This alteration is not simply due to differences in absorption as it occurs both with cortisone–glucose tolerance and i.v. glucose tolerance tests (Streeten *et al.*, 1965; Pozefsky *et al.*, 1965). Fasting and post-prandial blood glucose levels also rise with age. These findings probably are not clinically significant since they amount to no more than 0.1 mmol/l (2 mg/100 ml) and 0.2 mmol/l (4 mg/100 ml) respectively for each decade throughout adult life (O'Sullivan, 1972). The response to an oral dose of glucose, measured after 2 h, also alters with age. It rises by 0.06 mmol/l (1 mg/100 ml) per year of age and is higher in women than men (usually by 0.6 mmol/l or 10 mg/100 ml).

The metabolic clearance rate of insulin and its delivery into the system under resting conditions seems unchanged. No change in sensitivity to insulin has been noted with age.

Five per cent of all cases of diabetes are diagnosed between birth and 20 years. This contrasts sharply with the fact that 45% of cases are diagnosed over the age of 60 years (Pyke, 1968). Glycosuria is an unreliable diagnostic criterion in the elderly. In half the patients with clinically significant hyperglycaemia (>11.0 mmol/l), glycosuria is absent (Denham, 1972). Random mid-morning blood glucose estimations may be the most sensitive screening test in the elderly (Denham, 1972). It is essential that the diagnosis of diabetes in the elderly is not avoided but the alterations in the diagnostic parameters must be taken into account.

TREATMENT

The aim of therapy is to remove the symptoms (Table 6.1), prevent keto-acidosis and to restore the patient's resistance to infection. In the long term the serious sequelae, particularly those affecting the cardiovascular

Table 6.1   Clinical features of diabetes

---

(1) Thirst and polyuria
(2) Tiredness and malaise
(3) Weight loss (appetite is usually good)
(4) Skin complaints—pruritus vulvae/balantis
                    moniliasis
                    boils
(5) Cataract
(6) Visual upsets/retinopathy
(7) Peripheral vascular disease
(8) Nephropathy
(9) Neuropathy/autonomic dysfunction, e.g. impotence, nocturnal diarrhoea
(10) Glycosuria—may have noted that urine dries to a white stain

---

Maturity-onset diabetes usually has a much more insidious onset than juvenile diabetes.

and nervous systems, may be reduced or prevented. There is evidence that good control does reduce their incidence (Pirat, 1978).

In many instances the elderly diabetic can be well controlled on diet alone, or diet and an oral hypoglycaemic agent. The diet should be restricted in carbohydrate and should take into account the physical activity of the individual. Many elderly patients can have great difficulty in following a prepared diet sheet. The advice and help of an experienced dietitian can be invaluable in establishing a smooth routine. If the patient is obese it is essential that the weight be reduced and a 1000 kcal (10 g carbohydrate) diet can be used. Where the patient is not obese and is active then 1200–1400 kcal (120–140 g carbohydrate) per day may be more appropriate. It is very important that the diet should contain adequate fibre. This has been shown to reduce the absorption of saccharides (Jenkins *et al.*, 1977). Where diet fails to control the diabetes (persistent glycosuria or post-prandial glucose 8.3 mmol/l) then an oral hypoglycaemic agent should be introduced.

The oral hypoglycaemic agents fall into two groups—the sulphonylureas and the biguanides. The various drugs in the two categories are listed in Table 6.2. In the elderly the sulphonylureas are preferable to the biguanides, because of the very real risk of lactic acidosis when biguanides are used with any renal impairment (Luft *et al.*, 1978). The sulphonylureas act by stimulating the β cells of the pancreas so they are only effective where there is still some endogenous insulin production. The biguanides seem to exert their effect by increasing the peripheral uptake of glucose.

136

Table 6.2   Oral hypoglycaemic agents

Drug	Duration of action (h)	Site of metabolism	Active meta-bolites	Protein binding (%)
Sulphonylureas				
Glibenclamide	10–15	Liver Biliary excretion	–	99
Tolbutamide	6–10	Liver	–	95
Chlorpropamide	20–60	Liver Renal excretion	+	88–96
Biguanides				
Metformin	5–6	Renal excretion	–	0

Table 6.3   Studies of tolbutamide in relation to age

Study	Finding
Swerdloff *et al.* (1967)	Delayed and less profound drop in blood glucose
Sotaniemi and Huhti (1974)	Plasma protein binding correlates with age
Sotaniemi and Huhti (1974)	Plasma half-life unchanged
Miller *et al.* (1977)	Total plasma clearance and volume of distribution correlate with age

Table 6.4   Suggested schedule for oral hypoglycaemics in elderly patients

Glibenclamide	2.5–15 mg daily in one or two doses
Tolbutamide	0.5–3.0 g in three divided doses
Chlorpropamide	100–500 mg in one dose

Note: Patients initially responsive to sulphonylureas may, after some time, cease to respond. If this occurs then:
(a) check that patient is observing carbohydrate restriction and taking tablets;
(b) increase dose of sulphonylurea or change drug:
(c) add metformin 500 mg three times daily;
(d) if all else fails, transfer to insulin.

Glibenclamide and, to a lesser extent, tolbutamide, are the most commonly used preparations. Some clinicians still use chlorpropamide

Table 6.5   Side-effects of oral hypoglycaemic drugs

(A) Sulphonylureas
    (a) Allergic skin reactions and photosensitivity ⎱ Usually mild and
    (b) Gastrointestinal disturbance   ⎰   transient
    (c) Blood dyscrasias (agranulocytosis, leucopenia, and purpura)
    (d) Hypoglycaemia
    (e) Transient rise in alkaline phosphatase
    (f) Jaundice—usually cholestatic. Often preceded by rash
    (g) Water intoxication (chlorpropamide)
    (h) Facial flushing if alcohol taken (chlorpropamide)

(B) Biguanides
    (a) Lactic acidosis—carries a high mortality (50% +)
    (b) Dose-related gastrointestinal upsets—metallic taste, nausea, vomiting
    (c) Possibly increased cardiovascular deaths amongst those taking phen-
         formin

Table 6.6   Clinically important drug interactions with oral hypoglycaemic agents

Potentiating interactions	Antagonizing interactions
Phenylbutazone	Rifampicin
Oxyphenbutazone	Corticosteroids
Beta-blockers	Thiazide diuretics
Levodopa	
Aspirin	
Sulphonamides	
Alcohol	
Monoamine oxidase inhibitors	
Probenecid	
Chloramphenicol	
Dicoumarol (but probably not warfarin)	

because of the simplicity of once-daily dosage. However, it is widely felt that the risks of hypoglycaemia outweigh the consideration of dosage simplicity. Chlorpropamide has a half-life of more than 36 h and its plasma concentration varies widely due to genetically determined differences in biotransformation. At present a cloud hangs over tolbutamide following the findings of the University Group Diabetes Programme (1975). This suggested that therapy may well be associated with an increase in deaths from cardiovascular causes. However, the results from this study have been challenged and many physicians would continue to use this drug. Several studies of its handling with age have been carried

138

out and these are detailed in Table 6.3. Tolbutamide has genetically determined slow and fast acetylators (Scott and Poffenbarger, 1979).

Suggested schedules for the use of oral hypoglycaemic agents in the elderly are summarized in Table 6.4. Their side-effects are detailed in Table 6.5.

Clinically important drug interactions are detailed in Table 6.6.

INSULIN

Insulin is a low molecular weight two-chain polypeptide, synthesized by the β cells of the pancreas. It is carried on an α_1-globulin.

The choice of insulin regimen in the elderly needs careful consideration. Where the patient would be totally unable to manage an insulin regimen then the addition of metformin (a biguanide) to the diet and sulphonylurea regimen may be a more practical solution.

Most diabetic specialists now feel that a twice-daily regimen of short-acting insulin and the intermediate-acting isophane (IPH) provides the most effective and physiological control (Oakley *et al.*, 1976). Twice-daily regimens must be used if the daily insulin requirement is more than 40 units. The insulins recommended for this regimen are Actrapid or Leo neutral and porcine isophane (Retard). The isophane insulin enables the risk of hypoglycaemia to be reduced by using smaller doses of the short-acting insulin. If the older patient has difficulty in measuring a two-insulin mixture then a twice-daily fixed regimen of Monotard or Rapitard may be a good compromise. (For the compositions of these insulin preparations see Table 6.7.) Holman and Turner (1977) found that single daily injections of Ultralente gave good control in mild elderly diabetics. In single daily dose regimens Lente, Lentard, or Monotard insulins may also be used. Unfortunately, these regimens tend to give high morning blood glucose concentrations. A supplement of a short-acting insulin may be required (Actrapid or Semilente).

Whilst ideally the patient should be stabilized as an outpatient, this is not always feasible. It requires a great deal of supervision. It is therefore more likely that stabilization will be carried out in hospital. This gives the opportunity for good dietary advice, advice on foot care, stressing the importance of regular urine/blood tests, the care of syringes, choice of injection sites, preparation of the skin, measurement of insulin, etc. All patients should be given a card which states clearly that they are diabetic, and this should be carried with them at all times.

There are several unwanted effects of insulin therapy and these are noted in Table 6.8.

Table 6.7　Types of insulin

(HP)	Actrapid—short-acting porcine solution
(HP)	Leo neutral—short-acting porcine solution
(HP)	Retard (isophane)—intermediate-acting porcine solution (now known as Insulatard)
(HP)	Monotard MC—30% amorphous porcine; 79% crystalline porcine
(HP)	Rapitard MC—25% Actrapid MC: 75% crystalline bovine MC
	Lente—30% Semilente: 70% Ultralente
(HP)	Lentard MC—30% Semitard MC (porcine); 70% Ultratard MC (bovine)
	Semilente—short-acting beef suspension
	Ultralente—long-acting beef suspension

HP = High purified types.

Table 6.8　Complications of insulin therapy

(1) *Hypoglycaemia*
If frequent implies poor regimen
Administer oral/i.v. glucose
0.5–1.5 mg i.m. glucagon may be helpful
Features of overtreatment with insulin include lethargy, depression, night sweats, and morning headache
Recurrent nocturnal hypoglycaemia may cause rebound hyperglycaemia (Gale and Tattersall, 1979)

(2) *Insulin allergy*
May be due to poor skin preparation
Occasionally due to specific allergy to beast of origin

(3) *Lipodystrophy*
Occurs more often in women than men
Less common with the purified insulins

(4) *Insulin lumps*
Due to overuse of injection sites

(5) *Insulin resistance*
Often self-limiting
Use pork insulin
Very occasionally requires corticosteroids

There are several points to bear in mind when dealing with elderly diabetics:

(1) Age does not mean that treatment should be any less meticulous than in a younger patient.
(2) Management based solely on the presence or absence of glycosuria can be very misleading as elderly patients often do not exhibit glycosuria even when the blood glucose is above 11.0 mmol/l.

140

(3) Diabetic ketoacidosis carries a greater mortality in the elderly (Barnett *et al.*, 1962).
(4) Hyperosmolar coma can occur in the elderly, and serious potassium depletion can occur in the recovery phase unless careful monitoring is carried out.
(5) Hypoglycaemic symptoms in the elderly often occur at higher blood glucose levels—occasionally as high as 5–6 mmol/l.
(6) Hypoglycaemia in the aged can present as a cerebrovascular accident. This reverses completely with prompt therapy.
(7) Not infrequently glycosuria occurs in the elderly following a cerebrovascular accident. This is transient and requires no therapy.
(8) The treatment of diabetic coma is essentially the same in old and young patients.

Diabetes has an influence on the kinetics of other drugs. For instance, the absorption of i.m. penicillin is decreased in diabetic adults (Weinstein and Meade, 1976).

THYROID DISEASES

The thyroid gland synthesizes, stores, and secretes two iodinated amino acids—1-thyroxine (T_4) and 1-tri-iodothyronine (T_3). Control is by negative feedback via the hypothalamus and the pituitary gland. Circulating thyroid hormones are carried bound mainly to a globulin (thyroxine-binding globulin) and to a lesser extent by a pre-albumin and albumin (Chopra and Solomon, 1976). Changes in binding greatly influence the estimation of thyroid function tests (see Table 6.9).

Table 6.9   Changes in binding influencing thyroid function tests

(a) Interactions increasing thyroxine-binding globulin (TBG) capacity
    e.g. Oestrogens
(b) Decreasing TBG capacity due to competition for binding sites
    e.g. Phenytoin
       High-dose salicylates
       Clofibrate
(c) Decreased synthesis of TBG
    e.g. Testosterone
(d) Reduced levels of T_3 and T_4 without altering TBG
    e.g. Glucocorticoids
       Antithyroid drugs
(e) Increased total thyroxine concentrations
    e.g. Oestrogens

The main changes in the physiology of the thyroid gland associated with age are detailed in Chapter 1. Gregerman and Bierman (1974) showed a progressive decrease in T_4 disposal with age. Tri-iodothyronine decreases by 25–40% with age. In the main the age-related changes in the thyroid imply that lower doses of replacement thyroid hormones are required in old age.

Table 6.10   Clinical features of thyrotoxicosis

(1) *Skin*
Warm and moist
Heat intolerance
(Occasionally fever and hyperpyrexia)
Loss of hair
Nails recede from nail bed

(2) *Gastrointestinal system*
Usually weight loss although increased appetite (but appetite often reduced in elderly)
Diarrhoea
Thirst

(3) *Cardiovascular system*
Palpitations—tachycardia with large pulse volume
Short of breath on exertion
Angina
Sleeping pulse >80/min
* Atrial fibrillation—often resistant to digoxin
Systolic flow murmur
Systolic hypertension
* Unexplained congestive cardiac failure, especially in the elderly

(4) *Neuromuscular*
Tiredness, weakness
Tremor
Overactivity
Thyrotoxic myopathy (proximal)
Hyperactive reflexes
Occasionally myasthenia gravis
* Mental apathy

(5) *Skeletal*
Osteoporosis

(6) *Psychiatric*
* Irritable
Nervous
Insomnia
Rarely psychosis

* Common in elderly.

Table 6.11   Clinical features of hypothyroidism

(1) *Skin*
Dry skin and hair—hyperkeratosis over flexures
Cold intolerance
Facial puffiness
Occasionally vitiligo
Hypothermia

(2) *Gastrointestinal system*
Anorexia
Weight gain
* Constipation/faecal impaction
Rarely ascites

(3) *Cardiovascular system*
Diminished cardiac output
Low ECG complexes with flat T-waves
Pericardial effusion
Hyperlipoproteinaemia

(4) *Neuromuscular*
Apathy
Hallucinations—'myxoedema madness'
Hearing loss
Vertigo or rarely cerebellar ataxia
Median nerve entrapment
Peripheral neuropathy
Uveal effusions
Aches and pains and cramps
Prolonged reflex relaxation time

(5) *Respiratory system*
Alveolar hypoventilation
Pleural effusions

(6) *Haematology*
Anaemia—usually normoblastic but can present as
macrocytic or microcytic

* Common in elderly.

The two main thyroid diseases encountered in the elderly are firstly, thyrotoxicosis, which not infrequently presents as cardiac failure or apathy, and secondly myxoedema. The clinical features of both diseases are detailed in Tables 6.10 and 6.11 respectively. Thyroid carcinoma can also present in later life. However, this diagnosis is usually fairly straight-forward.

The interpretation of the laboratory tests of thyroid function (Table

6.12) varies slightly with age. Both serum thyroxine and to a more marked extent serum tri-iodothyronine show a drop with age. The normal values for serum thyroxine depend very much on the individual laboratory. Serum tri-iodothyronine would normally be within the range 1.0–2.6 mmol/l.

There is virtually no information regarding age-related changes in response to antithydroid drugs, and pharmacokinetic data are non-existent.

The therapeutic approaches to thyroid disease in the elderly are the same in the old as in the young.

Table 6.12   Thyroid function tests

(1) *Circulating thyroid hormones*
    (a) Serum thyroxine (T_4)
        Standard test
        Influenced by changes in binding proteins
        Can be influenced by drugs
        Slightly decreased with age
    (b) Serum tri-iodothyronine (T_3)
        Influenced by changes in binding
        More marked decline with age than T_4
    (c) Serum protein-bound iodine (PBI)
        Largely abandoned as a routine
    (d) Thyroid hormone-binding tests

(2) *Circulating levels of free thyroid hormones*
    (a) Free thyroxine
        Disagreement about levels
    (b) Free tri-iodothyronine
        Disagreement about levels
    (c) Calculated free thyroxine index

(3) *Dynamic tests of thyroid function*
    (a) [131]I uptake test
    (b) Tri-iodothyronine suppression test
    (c) TSH stimulation test

(4) *Tests of peripheral tissue response*
    (a) Tyrosine tolerance
    (b) Serum creatinine phosphokinase
    (c) Tendon reflex duration   } Relatively little clinical
    (d) Serum cholesterol   value
    (e) ECG
    (f) Cyclic AMP response to glucagon

Table 6.12   continued

---

(5) *Tests of hypothalamic pituitary function*
    (a) Thyroid-stimulating hormone immunoassay
        Slight increase in elderly
    (b) Thyrotrophin-releasing hormone test

(6) *Tests indicating cause of thyroid dysfunction*
    (a) Antithyroid antibodies
        Thyroglobulin antibodies
        Microsomal antibodies
        CA2 antibodies
        Cell surface antibodies
        Thyroid-stimulating antibodies
              Ultrasound
            ↗
    (b) Thyroid scan
            ↘
              Isotope
    (c) X-ray
    (d) Thyroid biopsy
    (e) Perchlorate discharge
    (f) Non-specific
        Plasma proteins
        ESR
        Flocculations

TREATMENT OF THYROTOXICOSIS

The mainstay of the treatment of thyrotoxicosis is carbimazole. (Other suitable preparations are detailed in Table 6.13.) It has a half-life of 7 h and has active metabolites. Normally the starting dose would be 30–40 mg daily in divided doses. Dividing the dose provides better control (Gwinup, 1978). This should be maintained until the patient becomes euthyroid (usually 6–8 weeks). The dose should then gradually be reduced to a maintenance dose of 5–15 mg daily. Effective control can be monitored by the clinical state (Mortimer *et al.*, 1977) and the serum thyroxine being within the range 51.5–142 mmol/l. It may eventually be possible to withdraw the drugs completely after about 2 years of treatment. However, if thyroid autonomy persists then radioiodine therapy or subtotal thyroidectomy need to be considered. The main problem with ^{131}I therapy is the high incidence of post-irradiation hypothyroidism (40–50% by 15 years). Many clinicians advocate small doses of thyroid replacement once the patient is euthyroid. In the elderly regular clinical assessment may well be preferable to unnecessary drug therapy.

If congestive cardiac failure has been a feature, then diuretics and possibly digoxin may be required until the thyrotoxicosis is under control. Thyrotoxic patients often require larger digoxin doses to obtain a given serum level: changes in absorption, distribution, metabolism, and elimination have all been implicated. Supraventricular arrhythmias in thyrotoxicosis may well respond better to propranolol than to digoxin, although again larger doses may be needed.

Table 6.13   Drugs for the treatment of thyrotoxicosis

	Initial dose (mg/day)	Maintenance dose (mg/day)
Carbimazole	40	5–15
Methimazole	24	3–9
Propylthiouracil	400	50–150
Methylthiouracil	400	50–150
Potassium perchlorate	800	200–400

Side-effects of these drugs include:
(a) Skin rashes
(b) Blood dyscrasias—agranulocytosis, thrombocytopenia
(c) Drug fever
(d) Loss of hair—particularly with carbimazole
(e) Arthralgia
(f) SLE syndrome.

TREATMENT OF MYXOEDEMA

Myxoedema can be one of the most satisfying diagnoses to make in an elderly patient. Care must be taken in the initial stages of therapy, especially where the patient has any evidence of ischaemic heart disease. The drug of choice is 1-thyroxine and this should be started in a dose of 0.05 mg daily for 2 weeks then 0.1 mg daily for the next 6 weeks. At the end of 2 months the patient's response should be assessed and TSH reassayed. It is rare for elderly patients to require more than 0.2 mg of thyroxine to control primary hypothyroidism. Many patients can be well managed on 0.15 mg daily. Because of the long half-life of thyroxine (up to 12 days in myxoedematous patients) the drug can be administered once daily, usually in the morning.

If ischaemic heart disease is present then propranolol 20 mg t.d.s. is required to prevent cardiac complications during the early stages of treatment.

The side-effects of thyroxine therapy are those of hyperthyroidism. Side-effects are often aggravated by caffeine. Weight reduction should also be encouraged.

Thyroid disease can influence how the body responds to other drugs. Huffmann *et al.* (1977) found that the increase in gastrointestinal motility associated with hyperthyroidism decreased the bioavailability of digoxin. The changes found in GFR also influence digoxin handling (Croxson and Ibbertson, 1975). Bradley *et al.* (1974) found a significant increase in GFR in hyperthyroid patients. There is some evidence to suggest that hepatic metabolism may also be influenced by thyroid disease. Antipyrine clearance is increased in hyperthyroidism and decreased in hypothyroidism (Eichelbaum, 1976). It has also been noted that the plasma concentration of propranolol is increased in hypothyroid patients (Feely and Stevenson, 1978).

OESTROGENS

The role of oestrogens in post-menopausal osteoporosis will be discussed in Chapter 7.

CORTICOSTEROIDS

Andres and Tobin (1977) summarized current knowledge about the effect of age on the hypothalamic–pituitary–adrenal axis. Plasma cortisol levels are unaffected by age, but the cortisol secretion rate and its rate of urinary excretion are reduced in the elderly. At least two studies have shown that cortisol half-life is substantially prolonged in older subjects. The clinical implications of the age changes in adrenal function and the response to glucocorticoid therapy in the elderly have not been studied.

REFERENCES

Andres, R. and Tobin, J. D. (1977) Endocrine systems. In Finch and Hayflicks (eds), *Handbook of the Biology of Ageing*, pp. 357–378. Van Nostrand Reinhold, New York.

Barnett, D. M. *et al.* (1962) Diabetic coma in persons over 60 years. *Geriatrics*, **17**, 327.

Bradley, S. E. *et al.* (1974) The thyroid and the kidney. *Kidney Int.*, **6**, 346.

Butterfield, W. J. H. (1964) Summary of the results of the Bedford Diabetes Survey. *Proc. Roy. Soc. Med.*, **57**, 196.

Chopra, I. J. and Solomon, D. H. (1976) Thyroid function tests and their alteration by drugs. *Pharmacol. Ther.*, Part Ci, 367.

Croxson, M. S. and Ibbertson, H. K. (1975) Serum digoxin in patients with thyroid disease. *Brit. Med. J.*, **3**, 566–8.

Denham, M. J. (1972) The value of random blood glucose determinations as a screening method for detecting diabetes mellitus in the elderly. *Age and Ageing*, **1**, 55.

Eichelbaum, M. (1976) Drug metabolism in thyroid disease. *Clin. Pharmacokinet.*, **1**, 339.

Feely, J. and Stevenson, I. H. (1978) The effect of age and the hyperthyroid state on plasma propranolol steady state concentration. *Brit. J. Clin. Pharmacol.*, **6**, 446P.

Gale, E. A. M. and Tatterssall, R. B. (1979) Unrecognized nocturnal hypoglycaemia in insulin treated diabetes. *Lancet*, **1**, 1049.

Gregerman, R. I. and Bierman, E. L. (1974) Ageing and hormones. In Williams (ed.), *Textbook of Endocrinology*, pp. 1059–70. Saunders, Philadelphia.

Gwinup, G. (1978) Prospective randomised trial of propylthiouracil. *JAMA*, **239**, 2457.

Holman, R. R. and Turner, R. C. (1977) Diabetes: the quest for basal normoglycaemia. *Lancet*, **1**, 469.

Huffmann, D. H. *et al.* (1977) Digoxin in hyperthyroidism. *Clin. Pharmacol. Ther.*, **22**, 533.

Jenkins, D. J. A. *et al.* (1977) Treatment of diabetes with guar gum. *Lancet*, **2**, 779.

Luft, D. *et al.* (1978) Lactic acidosis in biguanide treated diabetes. *Diabetologia*, **14**, 75.

Miller, A. K. *et al.* (1977) Effect of age on the pharmacokinetics of tolbutamide in man. *Pharmacologist*, **19**, 128.

Mortimer, C. H. *et al.* (1977) Thyrotoxicosis: relationships between clinical states and biochemical changes during carbimazole therapy. *Brit. Med. J.*, **1**, 138.

Oakley, W. G. *et al.* (1976) Insulin resistance. *Brit. Med. J.*, **2**, 134.

O'Sullivan, J. B. (1972) Age gradients in blood glucose levels: magnitude and clinical implications. *Diabetes*, **23**, 713.

Pirat, J. (1978) Diabetes mellitus and its complications: a prospective study, 1947–73. *Diabetic Care*, **1**, 168.

Pozefsky, I. *et al.* (1965) The cortisone–glucose tolerance test—the influence of age on performance. *Ann. Intern. Med.*, **63**, 998.

Pyke, D. A. (1968) The incidence and prevalence of diabetes. In W. G. Oakley, D. A. Pyke, and K. W. Taylor (eds), *Clinical Diabetes and its Biochemical Basis*, pp. 181–90. Blackwell Scientific Publications, Oxford.

Scott, J. and Poffenbarger, P. L. (1979) Pharmacogenetics of tolbutamide metabolism in humans. *Diabetes*, **28**, 41.

Sotaniemi, E. A. and Huhti, E. (1974) Half-life of intravenous tolbutamide in the serum of patients in medical wards. *Ann. Clin. Res.*, **6**, 146–54.

Streeten, R. D. *et al.* (1965) Reduced glucose tolerance in elderly human subjects. *Diabetes*, **14**, 579.

Swerdloff, R. S. *et al.* (1967) Influence of age on the intravenous tolbutamide test. *Diabetes*, **15**, 161–70.

University Group Diabetes Programme (1975) A study of the effects of hypoglycaemic agents on vascular complications in patients with adult onset diabetes (V). *Diabetes*, **24** (suppl. 1), 65.

Weinstein, L. and Meade, R. H. (1976) Absorption and excretion of intramuscular penicillin in diabetic patients. *Nature*, **192**, 987.

Chapter 7

Musculoskeletal disorders

The main problems to be considered in this chapter are rheumatoid arthritis, osteoarthritis, gout, polymyalgia rheumatica, Paget's disease, and osteoporosis.

The anatomical and physiological changes in the musculoskeletal system which accompany ageing are detailed in Chapter 1.

There are several general principles of therapy which apply to all the rheumatic disorders:

(1) Relieve the pain, stiffness, and swelling.
(2) Maintain the function of the joints.
(3) Try to prevent deformity.
(4) Consider the morale of the patient. Nothing is so dispiriting as constant pain which persists indefinitely.
(5) Remember that drugs are only one aspect of the therapeutic approach to these disorders. Other aspects of treatment such as surgery, occupational therapy, physiotherapy, rest, and exercise all have important roles to play.
(6) Educate the patient and his or her family regarding what to expect from the disease and the therapy.

Perhaps almost more than in any other aspect of medicine the therapy must be tailored to the individual's requirements. The doctor does not know which tablets are the most effective but the patient does—ask him.

Rheumatoid arthritis

This disease is complex and variable, both in time-span and severity. It not infrequently starts late in life. Although there are basic guidelines, each case must be assessed individually (Hart and Huskisson, 1972).

There are two main groups of drugs used in the treatment of rheumatoid arthritis. Firstly, the non-steroidal anti-inflammatory agents. These drugs act by inhibiting the production or action of the local pain-response mediators (McQueen, 1973). The second group contains drugs which seem to influence the disease process itself, e.g. gold, D-penicillamine, chloroquine, immunosuppressants, and corticosteroids.

This second group is used where there is no response to first-line therapy.

The choice of drug in any given situation is governed by several factors. These are summarized in Table 7.1. The main drugs are detailed in Table 7.2.

Table 7.1   Choice of drug in rheumatic disease

(1) Disease process
  (a) Acute active disease (e.g. acute gout or severe active rheumatoid)—a highly potent anti-inflammatory analgesic is required, e.g. phenylbutazone or indomethacin.
  (b) Degenerative arthritis with intermittent pain—a simple analgesic is required.
  (c) Severe pain associated with degenerative arthritis—this may require a more potent analgesic such as phenylbutazone.

(2) Activity of disease:
  Where despite anti-inflammatory drugs such as phenylbutazone the arthritis is progressing, then gold, etc., or corticosteroids must be considered.

(3) What is effective for the individual patient?

(4) Presence or absence of risk factors (see Note below)

(5) Side-effects of drug and interactions with existing therapy

Note

Risk factor	*Drug to be avoided or used with extreme caution*	
Age	Phenylbutazone:	Blood dyscrasias
		Congestive cardiac failure
	Codeine:	Severe constipation
	Corticosteroids:	Osteoporosis with crush fractures, especially in elderly females
Heart disease	Corticosteroids	⎫
(CCF and	ACTH	⎬ Fluid retention
Hypertension)	Phenylbutazone	⎭
Asthma	Aspirin: if it produces wheeze	
Dermatitis	Gold	
Psoriasis	Chloroquine	
Peptic ulcer	All antirheumatic drugs	
Severe hepatic/ renal impairment	Increased risk of toxicity, especially of gold and phenylbutazone	
Diabetes	Corticosteroids may aggravate diabetic control	
Anticoagulants	Salicylates	
	Phenylbutazone and oxyphenbutazone	

Table 7.2   Drugs in the treatment of rheumatic disease

Drug type	Dose (daily)	Route of elimination	Side-effects
(1) *Analgesic*			
Salicylates	0.6–1 g 4-hourly	Hepatic metabolism	Gastrointestinal symptoms
		Renal excretion	Occult gastro-intestinal bleeding, occasionally causing anaemia
			Tinnitus
			Asthma
Paracetamol	1–1.5 g 3–6 hourly	Hepatic metabolism	Hepatic necrosis
		Renal excretion	Constipation
			Nausea and vomiting
(2) *Anti-inflammatory drugs*			
Salicylate	As above	Antacids concomitantly reduce efficacy	
Phenylbutazone	200–400 mg t.d.s. with food	Hepatic metabolism	Gastrointestinal discomfort
		Renal excretion	Fluid retention
		Active metabolites	Skin reactions
			Blood dyscrasias
			Goitre
			Headache
			Vertigo
			Tinnitus
Indomethacin	25–50 mg t.d.s. with food	Hepatic metabolism	Gastrointestinal discomfort
	100 mg nocte	Enterohepatic circulation	Headache/cerebral sensations
		Renal excretion	Vertigo
			Tinnitus
Sulindac	100–200 mg b.d. with food	Sulphide metabolite	Gastrointestinal upset
			Headache
Propionic acid derivatives			
Ibuprofen	200–400 mg t.d.s. with food	Hepatic metabolism	Usually well tolerated
			Mild gastrointestinal upset
			Rash
			Rarely: headache, vertigo, tinnitus

Table 7.2   continued

Drug type	Dose (daily)	Route of elimination	Side-effects
Naproxen	375–750 mg either as one or two daily doses	Hepatic metabolism Renal excretion	As for ibuprofen
Fenoprofen	300–600 mg q.d.s. with food	Hepatic metabolism	As for ibuprofen
(3) *Drugs influencing the disease process*			
Gold (sodium aurothomalate)		Slow renal excretion	Blood dyscrasias Fever Skin rashes/dermatitis Mouth ulcers Haemorrhage (give dimercaprol) Pulmonary reactions Proteinuria Haematuria
Chloroquine	250 mg daily initially; 200 mg maintenance	Hepatic metabolism Renal excretion	Rashes and psoriasis Hair colour changes Leucopenia Peripheral neuropathy Ocular upsets*
D-penicil-lamine	125–250 mg Increasing to a maximum of 750 mg	Hepatic metabolism Renal excretion	Gastrointestinal upset Metallic taste Blood dyscrasias Haematuria/protein-uria Nephrotic syndrome Myasthenia gravis
(4) *Corticosteroids*			
Prednisolone { 2 mg 8-hourly 5 mg nocte		Hepatic metabolism	Electrolyte upsets Gastrointestinal upset Osteoporosis Crush fractures HPA suppression

* *Ocular upsets with chloroquine*
  (a) Deposition of the drug in the cornea causing haziness, photophobia, halos.
  (b) Degenerative fundal changes.

152

Salicylates

Salicylates have several actions (Lim, 1966). They inhibit prostaglandins, decrease the sensitivity of the pain receptors to bradykinins (Vane, 1974) and decrease the action of the lymphokinins (Morley, 1975). Importantly, from the viewpoint of side-effects, they also prolong bleeding time and inhibit platelet function. Salicylates cause almost daily occult faecal blood loss: this can lead to iron deficiency anaemia in the elderly in whom dietary iron is already marginal (Davies, 1977).

There is no evidence that salicylate binding is altered with age (Wallace *et al.*, 1976). Castleden *et al.* (1977) found that age did not influence salicylate absorption.

In the main, thee is no advantage to using other than simple soluble aspirin in doses of 0.6–1.0 g every 3–4 h with food, aiming for a therapeutic level of 15–30 mg/100 ml. It is feasible to administer higher doses, but few patients tolerate more than 5 g daily because of tinnitus and anorexia. With high doses of aspirin the metabolic pathways are very nearly saturated and small changes in the dose can result in very large changes in the plasma concentrations (Gibson *et al.*, 1976).

It is important to remember that many patients taking salicylates suffer from varying degrees of dyspepsia. Many take antacids (not necessarily prescribed by their doctor). The renal excretion of salicylate is increased with the alkalinization of the urine following antacid ingestion. The therapeutic levels can thus be reduced (Levy *et al.*, 1975). Corticosteroids taken at the same time as salicylates decrease the salicylate levels by increasing their metabolism. This may prevent therapeutic levels being reached (Bardare *et al.*, 1978). If the dosage of corticosteroids is reduced without careful note being taken of the salicylate levels, rebound toxicity can occur (Klineberg and Miller, 1965).

Pyrazoles—phenylbutazone, oxyphenbutazone

These drugs act by inhibiting prostaglandin synthesis, uncoupling oxidative phosphorylation, and decreasing the ATP-dependent biosynthesis of mucopolysaccharide sulphates in cartilage. They are also midly uricosuric.

There is diversity of opinion regarding the half-life of phenylbutazone in the elderly, with studies showing both an increase and a decrease in half-life (O'Malley *et al.*, 1971; Triggs *et al.*, 1975). Although Crooks *et al.* (1976) found a significant decrease in the clearance of phenylbutazone in elderly subjects (86 ml decreasing to 65 ml/h), Triggs *et al.* (1975) reported that plasma clearance was unaffected by age.

Phenylbutazone can cause severe problems in the elderly by the retention of salt and water (reducing urinary volume and increasing plasma volume), precipitating cardiac failure. It is highly protein-bound with a low volume of distribution. Phenylbutazone is thus a prime candidate for binding site displacement by drugs which bind to the same albumin site, e.g. warfarin and tolbutamide. Albumin binding also decreases with age (Wallace *et al.*, 1976).

The most serious risk with phenylbutazone therapy is that of bone marrow depression. Inman (1977) found that the haematological abnormalities were more common in women over the age of 65 years. The main haematological problems are agranulocytosis (usually within 3 months of starting therapy), aplastic anaemia (more often after at least 1 year of therapy) (Fowler and Faragher, 1977) or thrombocytopenia. All patients receiving this group of drugs should be warned to report any sore throat, rash, or fever to their doctor.

The maximum dosage should not be more than 200–400 mg daily in divided doses.

Indomethacin

This is a highly effective antipyretic and analgesic drug (Hart and Boardman, 1964). It inhibits the production of prostaglandins, uncouples oxidative phosphorylation in both the cartilage and hepatic mitochondria and inhibits the motility of the polymorphonuclear leucocytes.

Traeger *et al.* (1973) found a significant prolongation of the half-life of indomethacin in the elderly. Binding displacement reactions do not readily occur with indomethacin as, despite being highly protein-bound, it has a very large volume of distribution (Vessel *et al.*, 1975).

Some of its side-effects are dose-related—particularly headaches and unpleasant cerebral sensations. Brooks *et al.* (1975) found some evidence that the incidence of these side-effects was increased when aspirin was given at the same time. There is value in giving probenecid with indomethacin. This inhibits excretion and raises the plasma levels but does not increase the incidence of toxic reactions. Indeed Baber *et al.* (1978) found the incidence of side-effects to be less during the concomitant administation of probenecid.

Other side-effects are detailed in Table 7.2. The normal dosage is 25–50 mg administered with food up to thrice daily. Where morning stiffness is a problem, indomethacin either 75–100 mg nocte orally or 100 mg nocte by suppository is well tolerated and extremely effective.

154

Sulindac

This is less toxic than indomethacin. It is metabolized in the gut and the sulphide metabolite produces its clinical effect. The metabolite has a half-life of 18 h, making twice-daily administration effective. This is useful in the elderly, allowing simplification of dosage schedules.

Propionic acid derivatives

There are numerous members of this group. With the exceptions of naproxen and fenoprofen, most are less effective than aspirin, although better tolerated (Hart *et al.*, 1978). They are used as aspirin substitutes, but they should not be given with aspirin as aspirin may reduce their plasma levels. They also have the advantage of not interfering with anti-coagulants since they use different binding sites.

Ibuprofen is effective and well tolerated in mild cases in doses of up to 1200 mg. In the United States double this dose is used with great benefit (and more toxicity) in severe rheumatoid arthritis.

Naproxen has a long half-life (10–17 h) enabling satisfactory twice-daily administration.

Flufenamic and mefenamic acids

These frequently cause diarrhoea (which can be severe) and have no compensating advantages. Their use is not often indicated in the elderly.

Other drugs

There are also several drugs used in the treatment of rheumatoid arthritis which exert some undefined influence on the disease process itself. These drugs are gold, chloroquine derivatives, immuno-suppressants, and D-penicillamine. Only brief mention will be made of them here as it is felt that their use should be confined to specialist centres.

They are used in active progressive erosive cases but not in advanced chronic disease. The treatment is aimed at producing and maintaining a remission. Long courses of therapy are usually needed (Huskisson, 1978). A non-steroidal analgesic may be required at the same time. It is important to avoid combinations of drugs with similar side-effects, e.g. gold and phenylbutazone.

Gold. This heavy metal has been used to treat arthritis for 50 years. Its clinical usefulness was established in 1961 (Research Subcommittee of the Empire Rheumatism Council Report). Considerable changes have taken place in its administration (Gottlieb, 1977). It is usually given by injection although an oral gold preparation is available (Finkelstein *et al.*, 1976). The most common preparation is sodium aurothiomalate (dosage schedule Table 7.3). It has a half-life of 5–6 days. At present there is uncertainty about the value of serum gold estimations. Blood counts are useful as eosinophilia may precede a toxic reaction. The toxic effects are detailed in Table 7.2. As soon as the ESR starts to decline the dose should either be reduced or more widely spaced. It is ESSENTIAL that urinalysis for haematuria and proteinuria be done before each injection.

Table 7.3   Gold administration (this drug is best used in specialist centres)

Dose schedule
   10 mg i.m. weekly
   Increase by 10 mg weekly to a weekly maximum of 50 mg
   When ESR starts to fall either reduce dose or increase dose interval to 2–4
      weeks

Monitoring toxicity
   Do urinalysis before each injection
   Monitor blood count:
      white cells
      platelets
      eosinophils
   Discontinue at first sign of toxicity

Chloroquine derivatives. In most instances a course of 10–12 months' therapy is given. Side-effects (Table 7.2) are common. Regular ophthalmological examination is essential for the early detection of toxic eye complications.

D-penicillamine. The mode of action of this drug is still not understood. Its clinical use is similar to that of gold. Although side-effects are more common they are less severe than with gold (Table 7.2). The dosage schedule is 125–250 mg increasing every 1–3 months to a maximum of 750 mg. Improvement is slow to appear. At least 6 months must elapse after gold therapy before D-penicillamine is given, or the incidence of adverse reactions rises dramatically (Dodds *et al.*, 1980).

Table 7.4   Activities of corticosteroids

The activities of the glucocorticoids are basically anti-insulin. Has a circadian rhythm. Highly protein-bound.

 (1) Catabolic effect on protein with increased nitrogen excretion
 (2) Increase hepatic glycogen
 (3) Promote gluconeogenesis
 (4) Stimulate synthesis of hepatic enzymes
 (5) Stimulate mobilization of free fatty acids
 (6) Anti-inflammatory activity via actions on microvasculature
 (7) Impede endothelial stickiness and diapedesis
 (8) Produce lysis of lymphoid tissue—impair cellular mediated immunity
 (9) Influence distribution and excretion of body water
(10) Personality/psychiatric upsets
(11) Depress hypothalamic–pituitary axis
(12) Pharmacokinetics:
      cortisol half-life 90 min; prednisolone 2.1–3.5 h
      90% cortisol protein-bound
      hepatic metabolism
      urinary excretion of inactive glucuronide metabolites

Corticosteroids and ACTH

Initially the explanation for the effectiveness of corticosteroids in rheumatoid arthritis was the lysosomal stabilization theory (Weissmann and Thomas, 1964). This, however, does not satisfactorily explain everything. Corticosteroids have more effect on the inflammation than the actual course of the disease. Their pharmacokinetics are detailed in Table 7.4.

The use of these drugs carries significant problems. If more than 7.5 mg daily prednisolone is given for any more than a few weeks Cushingoid features can appear. Other side-effects are summarized in Table 7.2. It is therefore the aim to use not more than 2 mg prednisolone 8-hourly or 5 mg prednisolone nocte where morning stiffness is a problem.

ACTH has similar problems. Steroids (prednisolone 10–40 mg) can also be used for localized joint injection (Fitzgerald, 1976).

Osteoarthritis

The main symptoms of osteoarthritis are those of pain, stiffness, muscle weakness, and cramps. Pain from a joint is often referred to an associated muscle or a neighbouring joint. The classical illustration of this is hip pain referred to the knee. Fortunately, although degenerative changes occur in us all, symptoms are much less common. There are several clinical presentations requiring different therapeutic approaches (Haslock, 1976—see Table 7.5).

Treatment usually revolves round a combination of rest and exercise with appropriate analgesics. The analgesics are either simple analgesics or non-steroidal anti-inflammatory drugs (particularly useful in arthritis of the hip and cervical spine).

Table 7.5   Clinical groupings in osteoarthritis

---

(1) Pain when immobile

                      analgesics
                 ↗
If disturbing sleep
                 ↘
                     bed cradle
    Mild analgesic as required

(2) Pain when weightbearing (e.g. standing)
    Programmed rest/exercise
    Analgesics

(3) Pain when moving
    Exercises
    Analgesics
    Surgery

Anti-inflammatory analgesics are often more beneficial than simple analgesics.

If there is a psychogenic overlay antidepressants may help.

Again drugs are not the complete answer. Patient education, physiotherapy, occupational therapy, and surgery, particularly for osteoarthritis of the hip, all have substantial contributions to make to the satisfactory care of the patient.

Polymyalgia rheumatica

This disease is strongly associated with temporal arteritis. They are probably different expressions of one disease process—an arteritis (Myles, 1975). Both diseases virtually only occur in old people. The clinical features of polymyalgia rheumatica are detailed in Table 7.6. Prednisolone is usually dramatically effective (Hart, 1975a), although analgesics may also be needed. Treatment for polymyalgia rheumatica should start with prednisolone 15 mg per day, aiming to control symptoms and reduce the

158

Table 7.6 Clinical features of polymyalgia rheumatica

 (1) More common in women than men
 (2) Pain/stiffness in neck/shoulder (very occasionally in pelvis)
 (3) Stiffness more marked in morning
 (4) Headache/painful areas over head
 (5) Malaise
 (6) Low-grade pyrexia
 (7) Very high ESR
 (8) Occasionally mild anaemia
 (9) Temporal artery biopsy will be diagnostic in 50% of cases
(10) Trial of steroids virtually always diagnostic

ESR to normal (Hart, 1975a). The dose should be reduced by 2.5 mg every 3 months over the first year, then by 0.5 mg monthly to the lowest dose for symptom control.

In temporal arteritis prednisolone should be started immediately at 40 mg daily reducing to 10 mg daily over 1 year then by 1 mg increments to the lowest controlling dose. If eye, cranial, or temporal symptoms occur in polymyalgia rheumatica there is a real threat of blindness so the higher 40 mg schedule must be started immediately (Hart, 1975b).

Polymyositis

Corticosteroids will improve the muscle weakness in most patients. Treatment is usually started with prednisolone 60 mg daily with rapid reduction to 5–15 mg daily after initial symptom control. Relapse is common if treatment is stopped in less than 2–3 years. Immunosuppressant drugs can be useful for their steroid-sparing effect.

BONE DISORDERS

Osteoporosis

Osteoporosis is loss of bone, the residual bone being normal. There are several causes of secondary osteoporosis (Table 7.7). Most cases are of primary osteoporosis in post-menopausal women. Between the ages of 50 and 70 years osteoporosis is almost exclusively a disease of women, but by 70 years males start to succumb. The biochemistry (calcium, phosphate, and alkaline phosphatase) is normal. The main clinical features are summarized in Table 7.8. (The reader is also recommended a review article by Dent and Watson, 1966).

Pain is not usually a feature until there has been a fracture. The com-

Table 7.7   Causes of secondary osteoporosis

Generalized:	Hyperthyroidism
	Excessive adrenocorticosteroids
	Heparin osteoporosis
	Malabsorption syndromes
Localized:	Disuse or immobilization
	Sudeck's atrophy
	Rheumatoid arthritis

Table 7.8   Clinical features of osteoporosis

(1) *Vertebral compression*
Kyphosis
Loss of height
Back pain
Angulation of ribs producing skin folds

(2) *Susceptibility to fractures*

(3) *X-ray findings*
Due to decrease in bone mass $\begin{cases} \text{Cortical thickness} \downarrow \\ \text{Trabeculation} \downarrow \end{cases}$
Increased contrast between vertebral bodies and end-plates
'Codfish' vertebrae
Increased longitudinal trabeculation
Schmorl's nodes due to herniation of nucleus pulposus into the vertebral body
Decreased bone in femur/metatarsals/metacarpals

(4) *Bone microscopy is normal*

mon sites for fracture are the lower forearm, the neck of femur (a significant cause of mortality and morbidity in elderly women), and compression fractures of the lower thoracic and lumbar vertebrae (these may necessitate bed rest in the acutely painful stage).

The treatment of osteoporosis is at best controversial and unsatisfactory. No specific therapy has been proven to increase bone mass. Calcium supplements (1 g elemental calcium) combined with 1000 units of vitamin D daily have been tried in an effort to raise the serum calcium and prevent the nocturnal increase of parathyroid hormone and its resorptive action on bone (Ingham, 1974). However, elderly women tend to absorb calcium poorly. Even where absorption has been increased by a small dose of vitamin D, much of the extra calcium is merely excreted via the kidneys (Marshall and Nordin, 1977).

Fluoride has also been tried in doses of 40–60 mg daily (Jowsey *et al.*, 1972) in an attempt to increase bone formation. This has doubtful clinical value and fluoride has frequent side-effects.

Other suggestions have included anabolic steroids, calcitonin, and oestrogens. All have been tried alone and in combinations. Nordin *et al.* (1980) showed that combinations of calcium, oestrogen/norethisterone and vitamin D/vitamin D metabolite were beneficial in treating osteoporosis. However, the use of long-term hormone therapy is not un-controversial, having been implicated in the aetiology of cancer of the breast and uterus (Weiss, 1975).

Osteoporosis is thus one of the diseases where prevention is much much better than cure (Editorial, 1978). The preventive measures suggested are:

(1) adequate dietary calcium (800–1000 mg daily);
(2) regular exercise maintained throughout life (stimulates osteoblasts);
(3) at-risk patients proffered prophylactic calcium;
(4) bed rest kept to a minimum throughout adult life.

Paget's disease of bone

This disorder affects 10% of the population by the age of 80 years. The skeletal involvement is patchy. The areas most commonly involved are the pelvis, lumbar spine, femur, tibia, clavicle, and skull. At the sites involved there is greatly increased bone turnover and the new bone is spongy and disorganized. The disease process seems to have spells of activity and quiescence. In the active phase the alkaline phosphatase is elevated although the calcium and phosphorus are normal. Surprisingly few elderly patients suffer from high-output cardiac failure which can occur in association with Paget's disease. Other clinical features are summarized in Table 7.9.

In painful phases analgesics are required. Severe pain may be due to sarcomatous change. This may necessitate narcotic analgesics if surgical intervention is not feasible.

Calcitonin can produce dramatic relief of bone pain and evidence of biochemical remission. Long-term therapy with calcitonin appears to be free from major side-effects but it requires daily intramuscular injections of 50–100 units and is extremely expensive. Calcitonin appears to suppress the disease transiently rather than cure it. On stopping treatment, biochemical markers drift back to pre-treatment levels but bone pain may remain controlled.

Table 7.9   Clinical features of Paget's disease of bone

---

(1) More males than females suffer

(2) Bone deformity/pain

                              headache
                          ↗
(3) Enlargement of skull
                          ↘
                              deafness

(4) Vertebral enlargement—kyphosis/paraplegia

(5) Malignant osteosarcoma/malignant osteoclastoma

(6) X-rays
     bone resorption
     thickened fluffy skull
     sclerotic vertebrae

(7) Cardiac enlargement when more than 30% of skeleton involved

---

Diphosphonates look promising in the treatment of Paget's disease. They cause a selective suppression of osteoclast numbers and activity. Disodium etidronate is normally given orally as 5 mg/kg daily for about 6 months, after which symptom suppression may last for several years. Defective mineralization can occur with prolonged high doses, but is unlikely at the above dose. Other diphosphonates currently under trial appear to have a larger therapeutic ratio and to act more rapidly.

In severe generalized osseous Paget's disease the cytotoxic agent mithramycin may be tried with benefit. It is very toxic and is only tried as a last resort (Mundy and Raisz, 1974).

It must be re-emphasized that the vast majority of patients require no therapy at all.

Gout

Gout results from an abnormality in urate metabolism causing sustained high serum urate levels. In the majority of cases this is due to under-secretion following on an isolated defect in the renal handling of urate. A few cases of gout result from overproduction of urate. Drug therapy in gout falls into three main subdivisions:

(1) the treatment of the acute attack;
(2) the prevention of further acute episodes;
(3) dissolution of tophi.

Treatment of the acute attack

This consists of the prompt administration of an effective anti-inflammatory agent as early in the attack as possible: e.g. indomethacin 25–50 mg t.d.s. plus 100 mg by suppository at night. Phenylbutazone can also be very effective, but colchicine is probably not as effective, and is more toxic. Other possibilities are listed in Table 7.10. The effects of age on phenylbutazone and indomethacin handling have been discussed above.

When all else fails in the acute attack it may be necessary to resort to corticosteroids in initial doses of prednisolone 30 mg daily, reducing by 5–10 mg daily.

Table 7.10   Drug treatment of the acute attack of gout

Drug	Dosage schedule	Elimination	Side-effects
Indomethacin	25–50 mg t.d.s. with food; 75–100 mg nocte; reduce dose as attack declines	Hepatic metabolism Enterohepatic circulation Renal excretion	Gastrointestinal upset Headaches Cerebral sensations Drowsiness Mental confusion Hearing upset Blood dyscrasias Peripheral neuropathy Eye upsets
Phenylbutazone	600–800 mg in three doses; reduce by 200 mg daily	Hepatic metabolism Renal excretion	Fluid retention Hypertension, vertigo, rashes Goitre Blood dyscrasias Hepatitis
Colchicine (degraded by light)	1 mg immediately; 0.5 mg 4-hourly till 6 mg max.	Hepatic metabolism Biliary/renal excretion	Abdominal pain Nausea, vomiting/ diarrhoea Peripheral neuritis Alopecia Blood dyscrasias
Naproxen	500–750 mg immediately then 250 mg 8-hourly	Hepatic metabolism Renal excretion	Gastrointestinal upset Asthma Proctitis if given rectally

Table 7.11 Drugs to normalize serum urate and to reduce tophi

Drug	Dosage schedule	Elimination	Side-effects
Probenecid	0.25 g b.d./t.d.s. for 1 week; increased to 1–2 g by 3 weeks	Hepatic metabolism	Gastrointestinal irritation Skin rash Headache Flushing Urinary frequency Nephrotic syndrome Hepatic necrosis Aplastic anaemia
Sulphinpyrazone	100 mg b.d. for a week; may increase to 300–600 mg	Hepatic metabolites Renal excretion	Gastrointestinal irritation Skin rash Fever
Benzbromarone	50 mg for 7 days; rising to 200 mg daily	Hepatic metabolism Renal excretion Active metabolites	Diarrhoea
Allopurinol	200 mg for 7 days; may increase to 400–600 mg	Hepatic metabolism Renal excretion	Rash Pruritus Fever Leucopenia Alopecia Hepatotoxicity Vertigo Gastrointestinal upsets Drowsiness Malaise Taste upset

Prevention of further acute episodes

This aspect of therapy is in two parts. Firstly, dietary education is needed to avoid high purine intake, reduce obesity, correct hyperlipoproteinaemia (Type IV) and maintain a high urinary output. The second line of attack is drug therapy, which should be reserved for patients with maintained high serum urate levels (9–11 mg/100 ml or 0.54–0.65 mmol/l), patients with tophi and those with frequent attacks.

There are two classes of urate-altering drugs: uricosuric agents, e.g.

probenecid; and the xanthine oxidase inhibitor allopurinol. Therapy with these drugs is detailed in Table 7.11. No studies of the effect of age on the handling of these drugs are available.

It is also worth remembering that many drugs can themselves produce arthralgia and other musculoskeletal side-effects. These are summarized in Table 7.12.

Table 7.12 Drugs which may produce musculoskeletal symptoms

Drug	Symptom complex
Procainamide Isoniazid Phenytoin	SLE syndrome
Isoniazid Sulphonamides Corticosteroids Pyrazinamide Ethionamide	Arthralgia
Diuretics Corticosteroids Carbenoxolone	Cramps
Diuretics Pyrazinamide Cytotoxic drugs	Gout
Corticosteroids	Bone necrosis
Anticonvulsants Antacids	Osteomalacia

REFERENCES

Baber, N. *et al.* (1978) The interaction between indomethacin and probenecid: a clinical and pharmacokinetic study. *Clin. Pharmacol. Ther.*, **24**, 298.

Bardare, M. *et al.* (1978) Value of monitoring plasma salicylate levels in treating juvenile rheumatoid arthritis. *Arch. Dis. Child.*, **53**, 381.

Brooks, P. M. *et al.* (1975) Indomethacin—aspirin interaction: a clinical appraisal. *Brit. Med. J.*, **3**, 69.

Castleden, C. M. *et al.* (1977) The effect of ageing on drug absorption from the gut. *Age and Ageing*, **6**, 138–43.

Crooks, J. *et al.* (1976) Pharmacokinetics in the elderly. *Clin. Pharmacokinet.*, **1**, 280–96.

Davies, D. M. (ed.) (1977) *Textbook of Adverse Drug Reactions*, p. 137. Oxford University Press, Oxford.

Dent, C. E. and Watson, L. (1966) *Postgrad. Med. J.*, **42**, 581.

Dodds, M. J. *et al.* (1980) Adverse reactions to D-penicillamine after gold toxicity. *Brit. Med. J.*, **280**, 1498.

Editorial (1978) Treatment of osteoporosis. *Brit. Med. J.*, **1**, 1303–4.

Finkelstein, A. E. *et al.* (1976) *Ann. Rheuma. Dis.*, **35**, 251.

Fitzgerald, R. H. (1976) Intrasynovial injection of steroids. *Mayo Clin. Proc.*, **51**, 655.

Fowler, P. D. and Farragher, E. B. (1977) Drug and non-drug factors influencing adverse reactions to pyrazoles. *J. Int. Med. Res.*, **5** (suppl. 2), 108.

Gibson, T. J. *et al.* (1976) Evidence that D-penicillamine alters the course of rheumatoid arthritis. *Rheumatol. Rehabil.*, **15**, 211.

Gottlieb, N. L. (1977) Chrysotherapy. *Bull. Rheum. Dis.*, **27**, 912.

Hart, F. D. (1975a) Inflammatory disease and its control in rheumatic disorders. *Brit. Med. J.*, **4**, 191.

Hart, F. D. (1975b) Visual complications of polymyalgia rheumatics. *Practitioner*, **215**, 763.

Hart, F. D. and Boardman, P. L. (1964) Indomethacin. *Practitioner*, **192**, 282.

Hart, F. D. and Huskisson, E. C. (1972) Pain patterns in the rheumatic disorders. *Brit. Med. J.*, **4**, 213.

Hart, F. D. *et al.* (1978) Non-steroidal anti-inflammatory agents. In F. D. Hart (ed.), *Drug Treatment of the Rheumatic Diseases*, p. 8. ADIS Press, Sydney.

Haslock, I. (1976) Medical treatment of osteoarthritis. *Clin. Rheum. Dis.*, **2**, 615.

Huskisson, E. C. (1978) Drugs which affect the rheumatoid disease process. In F. D. Hart (ed.), *Drug Treatment of the Rheumatic Diseases*, p. 44. ADIS Press, Sydney.

Ingham, J. (1974) Osteoporosis: its diagnosis and treatment. *Drugs*, **8**, 290.

Inman, W. H. (1977) A study of fatal bone marrow depression with special reference to phenylbutazone and oxyphenbutazone. *Brit. Med. J.*, **1**, 1500.

Jowsey, J. *et al.* (1972) Effect of combined therapy with sodium fluoride, UHD and calcium in osteoporosis. *Am. J. Med.*, **53**, 43.

Klineberg, J. R. and Miller, R. (1965) Effect of corticosteroids on blood salicylate concentrations. *JAMA*, **194**, 601.

Levy, G. *et al.* (1975) Decreased serum salicylate concentrations in children with rheumatic fever treated with antacids. *New Engl. J. Med.*, **293**, 323.

Lim, R. K. S. (1966) Salicylate analgesia. In Smith and Smith (eds), *The Salicylates: a Critical Bibliographic Review*. Wiley, New York.

McQueen, E. G. (1973) Anti-inflammatory drug mechanisms. *Drugs*, **6**, 104.

Marshall, D. H. and Nordin, B. E. C. (1977) The effect of 1α-hydroxyvitamin D3 with and without oestrogen on calcium balance in post-menopausal women. *Clin. Endocrinol.*, **7**, 159S.

Morley, J. (1975) *Proceedings of the Aspirin Symposium*, p. 19. Royal College of Surgeons.

Mundy, G. R. and Raisz, L. G. (1974) Drugs for disorders of bone. *Drugs*, **8**, 250.

Myles, A. B. (1975) Polymyalgia rheumatica and giant cell arteritis: a 7 year survey. *Rheumatol. Rehabil.*, **14**, 231.

Nordin, B. E. C. *et al.* (1980) The treatment of spinal osteopororis in post-menopausal women. *Brit. Med. J.*, **280**, 451–4.

O'Malley, K. *et al.* (1971) Determinants of anticoagulant control in patients receiving warfarin. *Brit. J. Clin. Pharmacol.*, **4**, 309–14.

Research Subcommittee of the Empire Rheumatism Council (1961). *Ann. Rheum. Dis.*, **20**, 315.

Traeger, A. *et al.* (1973) Zur Pharmakokinetik von Indomethacin bei alten Menschen. *Zeit. Altersforsch.*, **27**, 151–5.

Triggs, E. J. *et al.* (1975) Pharmacokinetics in the elderly. *Eur. J. Clin. Pharmacol.*, **8**, 55–62.

Vane, J. R. (1974) In Robinson and J. R. Vane (eds), *Prostaglandin Synthetase Inhibitors*, p. 159. Raven Press, New York.

Vessel, E. S. *et al.* (1975) Failure of indomethacin and warfarin to interact in normal human volunteers. *J. Clin. Pharmacol.*, **15**, 486.

Wallace, S. *et al.* (1976) Factors affecting drug binding in plasma of elderly patients. *Brit. J. of Clin. Pharmacol.*, **3**, 327–30.

Weiss, N. S. (1975) Risks and benefits of oestrogen use. *New Engl. J. Med.*, **293**, 1200–1.

Weissmann, G. and Thomas, L. (1964) The effects of corticosteroids on connective tissue and lysosomes. *Rec. Prog. Horm. Res.*, **20**, 215.

Chapter 8

Gastrointestinal problems

In the main, the treatment of gastrointestinal problems in the elderly follows the same basic principles that would be applied to younger subjects. They will therefore only be considered briefly. It is also important to remember that many drugs can cause or aggravate gastrointestinal symptoms. The influence of gastrointestinal motility and disease on drug handling is discussed in Chapter 2.

HIATUS HERNIA

This is a relatively common finding which in most cases is asymptomatic. Where symptoms are present (due to oesophageal reflux) then medical treatment should be tried first as surgical intervention is not always satisfactory. The treatment schedule is:

(1) If the patient is obese, weight must be lost.
(2) Elevate the head of the bed. Propping the patient up on pillows is not successful, as it tends to raise the intra-abdominal pressure and aggravate the reflux.
(3) Similarly tight corsets and restrictive clothing should be avoided.
(4) Patients should avoid eating for at least 2 h prior to retiring at night.
(5) Bending should be avoided.
(6) Drug therapy. There are several therapeutic approaches which can be made. Gaviscon (an alginate–antacid) has been advocated. It produces a soft viscous layer of antacid on top of the gastric contents, thus protecting the oesophagus from gastric reflux (Stanciu and Bennet, 1974). Normal dosage is two tablets as required and nocte.

    Simple antacids may also be of benefit. They are usually administered p.r.n. but some people find considerable benefit from a regular daily schedule.

    Pyrogastrone has also been recommended—one or two tablets t.d.s. after food and two tablets at bedtime. However, this can cause severe problems in the elderly as it contains carbenoxalone.

    Cimetidine can be of great benefit. As discussed later, the dose in the elderly subject must be reduced. 200 mg 12-hourly is usually adequate. However, some patients need higher doses and 200 mg t.d.s. and 200–400 mg nocte may be required.

(7) Anticholinergic drugs should be avoided since they reduce gastric motility and emptying.

PEPTIC ULCER

The aims of therapy in the treatment of peptic ulcer are to:

(1) relieve the pain;
(2) heal the ulcer;
(3) delay or prevent recurrences of the ulcer;
(4) prevent the complications of peptic ulceration.

It is, however, essential that the same care should be taken to exclude neoplasm in the elderly as in the younger patient. Endoscopy or radiological examination is therefore essential.

The possible therapeutic choices (doses and side-effects) are summarized in Table 8.1. However, a few specific points about their application to the elderly patient need to be made.

Cimetidine is a specific competitive histamine H_2 antagonist (Brogden *et al.*, 1978). It is now widely used to accelerate the healing of duodenal and gastric ulcers. Most of the dose of cimetidine is excreted unchanged via the kidneys. It is therefore important that smaller doses be used in elderly subjects to compensate for the age-related decline in renal function. Mental confusion has been reported as a side-effect of cimetidine therapy in the elderly. This is thought to be due to high trough concentrations as a consequence of reduced glomerular filtration in the elderly. In the main, 200–300 mg 12-hourly given with food is adequate in elderly patients.

Carbenoxalone is also used to promote healing of peptic ulcers. However, due to its mineralocorticoid activity it produces severe side-effects, notably profound hypokalaemia. It is normally extensively protein-bound and has a low volume of distribution. Its albumin-binding is reduced in the elderly and its rate of elimination is prolonged (Hayes *et al.*, 1977). For these reasons lower doses are required in the elderly. In the main, it is best to avoid this preparation in elderly patients and, if necessary, use the deglycyrrhizinated licorice preparation Caved-S which is much better tolerated.

It is important that the simple aspects of treatment are not overlooked:

(1) stop smoking;
(2) avoid ulcerogenic drugs such as aspirin;

(3) avoid alcohol and coffee;
(4) avoid foods which provoke symptoms;
(5) ? role of anti-anxiety drugs.

Thirty to sixty per cent of ulcers heal in 4–6 weeks almost regardless of therapy (Langman, 1977). It is important to bear this in mind and to balance this fact against the risks of therapy.

Table 8.1   Drugs used in the treatment of peptic ulcer

Drug	Action	Dose	Side-effects
(A) *Antacids*			
Magnesium hydroxide	Neutralization of gastric juice	5–10 ml p.r.n.	Diarrhoea with magnesium salts
Aluminium hydroxide		One or two tablets p.r.n.	Constipation with aluminium salts
Calcium carbonate		Intensive hourly administration highly effective	Best avoided in the elderly
(B) *Cimetidine*	Inhibits secretion of gastric acid	200 mg 12-hourly in elderly (if renal function good may increase to 200 mg t.d.s. after meals and 400 mg nocte)	Mental confusion in the elderly Gynaecomastia
(C) *Carbenoxalone* (Common preparations: Pyrogastrone, Biogastrone)	Enhances mucus production ? Influences hydrogen ions ? Has antipepsin activity	One or two tablets t.d.s. after meals	Fluid retention Hypokalaemia Hypertension Alkalosis *Avoid* use with spironolactone
(D) *Caved-S*	? Influences mucus production ? Antispasmodic	Two tablets t.d.s. with water	As effective as cimetidine (Morgan *et al.*, 1978)
(E) *Bismuth preparations* Best avoided as they are only weak antacids and have been incriminated in producing encephalopathy.			

CONSTIPATION

Much laxative-taking by the elderly (indeed by most people) is totally unnecessary and is caused by an obsession with a daily bowel motion. It is important that this excessive consumption of laxatives be discouraged and healthier habits encouraged:

(1) bran with cereal or fruit at breakfast time and a high-residue diet;
(2) plenty of fluids;
(3) encourage physical activity;
(4) prompt attention to the call to stool.

Where laxatives are required, it is essential that they are used in the lowest effective dose for the shortest possible time. In cases of presbycolon of the elderly (Bank and Marks, 1977) indefinite laxative therapy may be required, but again the lowest effective dose should be used.

The various types of laxatives and their side-effects are summarized in Table 8.2. The response to each individual preparation is highly variable and the dose needs to be suited carefully to the particular patient.

Where there is faecal impaction small-volume phosphate or citrate enemas may be required initially.

In all cases an underlying physical cause must be excluded.

A high-residue diet is also important in the medical management of diverticulosis and diverticulitis (Brodribb, 1977).

Whilst it is important to remember that gastrointestinal disease can alter drug handling, it is also as well to note that drugs can provoke gastrointestinal disease. A brief resumé of this nook of the iatrogenic world is encapsulated in Figure 8.1.

Table 8.2   Laxatives

Group	Daily dose	Side-effects
(1) *Irritants*		
Anthraquinones		
Cascara	Avoid	Risk of habitual use
		Melanosis coli
Senna	0.5–2 g (effective in the elderly)	Skin rashes
		Alterations in bowel ganglia
Biscodyl	5–15 mg	Abdominal cramps
Phenolphthalein	} Avoid	
Castor oil		
(2) *Bulk producers*		
Seeds/gums, etc.		
Isogel	5–10 g — All suitable	Occasionally reduces calcium uptake
Normacol	5–10 g — for elderly	
Bran	1–4 g — subjects and	
Methycellulose	3–6 g — long-term use	Flatulence
(3) *Osmotic preparations*		
Magnesium compounds	Avoid	Hypermagnesaemia secondary to impaired renal function
Small volume enema	Can be initial therapy in severe constipation	
(4) *Lubricants*		
Liquid paraffin	Avoid	Lipid pneumonia
		Anal leakage
		Impaired uptake of fat-soluble vitamins
(5) *Wetting agents*		
Poloxalkol	Avoid	Anorexia
Dioctylsodium sulphosuccinate		Nausea and vomiting

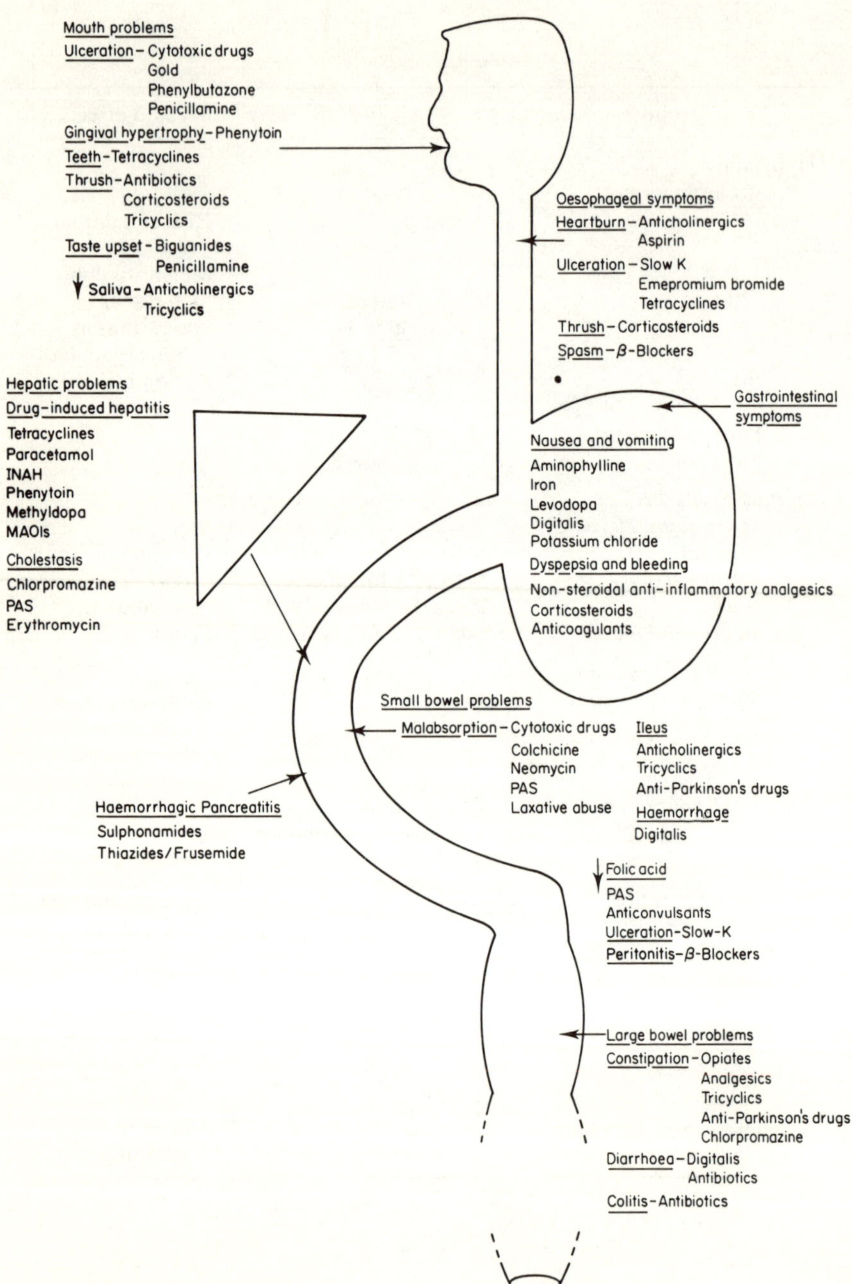

Fig. 8.1   Drug-induced/aggravated gastrointestinal disease

REFERENCES AND BIBLIOGRAPHY

Bank, S. and Marks, I. N. (1977) The etiology of constipation and diarrhoea in geriatric patients. *S. Afr. Med. J.*, **51**, 409.

Brodribb, A. J. M. (1977) The treatment of symptomatic diverticular disease with a high fibre diet. *Lancet*, **1**, 664.

Brogden, R. N. *et al.* (1978) Cimetidine: a review of its pharmacological properties and therapeutic efficacy in peptic ulcer disease. *Drugs*, **15**, 93.

Crowson, T. D. *et al.* (1976) Oesophageal ulceration associated with tetracycline therapy. *JAMA*, **235**, 2747.

Farquharson-Roberts, M. A. *et al.* (1970) Perforation of the small bowel due to Slow-K. *Brit. Med. J.*, **3**, 206.

Hayes, M. J. *et al.* (1977) Changes in the clearance and protein binding of carbenoxalone with age and possible relationship to adverse drug reactions. *Gut*, **18**, 1054.

Jick, H. and Porter, J. (1978) Drug-induced gastrointestinal bleeding (B.C.D.S.P.). *Lancet*, **2**, 87.

Keith, D. A. (1978) Side-effects of diphenylhydantoin. *J. Oral Surg.*, **36**, 206.

Kobler, E. *et al.* (1978) Drug-induced oesophageal ulceration. *Dtsch Med. Wochenschr.*, **103**, 1035.

Langman, M. J. S. (1977) Drugs in the treatment of gastric and duodenal ulcer. *Drugs*, **14**, 105.

Lelly, A. H. and Van Enter, C. H. J. (1970) Large-scale digitoxin intoxication. *Brit. Med. J.*, **3**, 737.

Milner, G. and Buckler, E. G. (1964) Adynamic ileus and amitriptyline. *Med. J. Aust.*, **1**, 921.

Morgan, A. G. *et al.* (1978) Cimetidine: an advance in gastric ulcer treatment? *Brit. Med. J.*, **2**, 1323.

Nakashima, Y. and Howard, J. M. (1977) Drug-induced acute pancreatitis. *Surg. Gynaecol. Obstet.*, **145**, 105.

Race, T. F. *et al.* (1970) Intestinal malabsorption due to colchicine. *Am. J. Med. Sci.*, **259**, 32.

Smith, E. R. and Goulston, S. J. M. (1975) Antibiotic-induced diarrhoea. *Drugs*, **10**, 329.

Smith, V. M. (1978) Association of aspirin with oesophageal disease. *South. Med. J.*, **71** (suppl.), 45.

Stanciu, C. and Bennet, J. R. (1974) Alginate–antacid in the reduction of oesophageal reflux. *Lancet*, **1**, 109.

Zfass, A. M. *et al.* (1970) Inhibitory β-adrenoreceptor activity in the distal oesophagus. *Am. J. Dig. Dis.*, **15**, 303.

Chapter 9

Respiratory disease

The changes in the anatomy and physiology of the respiratory system associated with ageing are detailed in Chapter 1. For a detailed text on the workings of the normal lung, the reader is referred to Murray (1976).

Chronic bronchitis and emphysema tend to become more common with advancing years. Late-onset asthma can be relentlessly progressive. The chance of dying in acute severe asthma rises with age: half of asthma deaths had their first attack of asthma after the age of 40 years (Macdonald *et al.*, 1976). In the main the treatment of these diseases is not greatly influenced by the age of the patient. As in all treatment an accurate diagnosis is essential to proper therapy. Most patients can be treated at home, but severe asthma, severe respiratory infections and respiratory failure necessitate urgent hospital admission.

The main diseases which will be considered here are asthma, chronic obstructive airways disease and respiratory failure.

ASTHMA

The principles of the treatment of asthma do not change with age. Patients with mild intermittent wheezing are best treated by aerosol β-agonist bronchodilators such as salbutamol or terbutaline. If this is inadequate then regular prophylaxis with aerosol steroids is needed. methyl xanthine and bronchodilators can have a useful adjuvant role but can rarely be the mainstay of treatment. If aerosol steroids do not control wheezing adequately then oral steroids are necessary. Their long-term use can bring the problem of osteoporosis, but failure to use adequate doses can and does cause years of unnecessary dyspnoeic misery. The main drugs used in treating asthma are outlined in Tables 9.1 and 9.2.

Acute severe asthma (status asthmaticus) is a medical emergency and should be dealt with by a specialist chest physician. A suggested regimen for the management of severe asthma is outlined in Table 9.3.

There are relatively few studies of the pharmacokinetics of these drugs in elderly subjects. There is some evidence (Piafsky *et al.*, 1977a) that age does not influence the elimination half-life or the apparent volume of distribution of theophylline. However, congestive cardiac failure did signifi-

174

cantly reduce the rate of plasma clearance of theophylline (Piafsky *et al.*, 1977b). In a recently published nomogram for intravenous theophylline,

Table 9.1   Drugs used in asthma

Drug	Type	Preparations	Dose	Side-effects
Bronchodilators				
Salbutamol	Selective β2-agonist (β1 at high doses)	Tablets	2–4 mg q.d.s.	Tremor Headache
		Inhaler	Two puffs	Tachycardia
		Solution	2 ml over 4 min q.d.s.	Nausea Vomiting
		Injection	250 μg 4-hourly	
Terbutaline	Selective β2-agonist	Tablets	5 mg t.d.s.	As above
		Inhaler	Two puffs	
		Solution	2–5 mg	
		Injection	200–500 μg 4-hourly	
Fenoterol	Selective β2-agonist	Inhaler	Two puffs	As above
Rimiterol	Selective β2-agonist	Inhaler	One to three puffs	As above
Orciprenaline	β2-agonist	Tablets	20 mg q.d.s.	Tremor
		Inhaler	Two puffs	Tachycardia
		Injection	500 μg	

α- and β-agonists such as ephedrine should be regarded as obsolete.

Theophylline ⎫
Aminophylline ⎭ Methylxanthine bronchodilators (see Table 9.2)

Drug	Type	Preparations	Dose	Side-effects
Regular prophylaxis				
Beclomethasone dipropionate	Corticosteroid	Inhaler	Three puffs t.d.s.	Hoarseness; oral thrush
Bisodium cromoglycate	—	Spinhaler or Inhaler	One capsule t.d.s. Two puffs q.d.s.	—

Notes:

(1) If patient does not respond to normal therapy, specialist advice should be sought immediately.

(2) Patients may be helped by taking their bronchodilator inhaler prior to an activity which normally produces breathlessness.

Table 9.2   Methylxanthine bronchodilators

Theophylline
200–800 mg twice daily, to give serum level 10–20 µg/ml
Marked variation in elimination—hepatic metabolism by demethylation
   oxidation
Clearance decreased with age
Clearance decreased by obesity, heavy coffee intake
Clearance decreased in CCF, pulmonary oedema, cor pulmonale, hepatic dis-
   ease
Clearance decreased by erythromycin
Clearance increased by smoking (>10 cigarettes per day)

Aminophylline (*theophylline ethylenediamine*)
225–900 mg twice daily, to give serum theophylline level 10–20 µg/ml
250–500 mg slow i.v. injection, then i.v. infusion (0.6 mg/kg/h)

Side-effects
Nausea, arrhythmias, excitation, insomnia, nightmares, convulsions

age was one of the variables (Jusko *et al.*, 1977). A dosage reduction of 25% was suggested in the elderly to maintain plasma levels in the therapeutic range (10–15 µg/ml). The patient's smoking history is important: Powell *et al.* (1978) found that it markedly increased the rate of theophylline clearance, requiring a dosage increase of 50% to compensate. Because of the increased incidence of cardiovascular disease in the aged, they are likely to be more susceptible to the toxic arrhythmias which can be produced by theophylline and related compounds. Extra care should therefore be taken in this situation to ensure that injections and infusions are not given rapidly. With regard to other drugs used in the treatment of asthma, no evidence at present exists for alterations in effect due specifically to age.

Many drugs used to relieve airways obstruction are administered by aerosol. It is essential that good aerosol technique is taught carefully and reinforced from time to time.

Simple lung function tests are also essential to assess the effectiveness of therapy. This is particularly so in patients admitted to hospital with severe asthma. Important diagnostic signs of ineffective treatment are failure of the peak expiratory flow rate to rise, failure of the pulse rate to drop below 100/min, persistent pulsus paradoxus and a normal PCO_2 (Macdonald *et al.*, 1976). It cannot be emphasized too strongly that severe asthma is a dire emergency which should be managed in hospital, preferably under the care of a specialist respiratory physician.

Table 9.3 Management of acute severe asthma

Immediate treatment
Measure blood gases and peak expiratory flow rate (PEFR)
Loading doses of:
  aminophylline 6 mg/kg i.v. slowly (unless currently taking slow-release
    theophyllines);
  hydrocortisone 500 mg i.v.
Nebulized salbutamol 10 mg or terbutaline 10 mg
Oxygen 35% via mask if tolerated by patient, if pCO_2 not raised

Continuation treatment
Intravenous infusion of 0.5 l normal saline 6-hourly, containing:
  aminophylline 4 mg/kg
  hydrocortisone 500 mg
Nebulized bronchodilator (as above) repeated 4-hourly
Oxygen as above
Monitor:
  PEFR 6-hourly
  Pulse
  Blood gases if no prompt clinical response
  Serum K^+

Further management
After 48 h, discontinue i.v. infusion if clinical, PEFR and pulse responses all
good. Then start oral prednisolone 10–15 mg 6-hourly:
(a) if pulse or PEFR response inadequate, continue infusion and remeasure
    blood gases;
(b) if any deterioration, consider artificial ventilation early.
Taper down oral steroids slowly and aim to discharge uncomplicated case in 7–10
days.

Note:
Asthma can kill: if in doubt, *overtreat*.

CHRONIC BRONCHITIS AND
EMPHYSEMA

These conditions are common in older patients, largely due to a lifetime
of cigarette smoking. It is never too late to stop smoking. Whilst the
damage done to the lungs does not reverse, it at least removes a continuing insult which is making matters worse.

In health the respiratory tree is effectively sterile below the vocal cords
but in mucopurulent bronchitis organisms, especially *H. influenzae* and
Strep. pneumoniae, are found. Secondary infection by these organisms
usually follows an upper respiratory tract infection. The choice of anti-

biotic is one of the broad-spectrum oral preparations such as ampicillin, amoxycillin, cotrimaxazole, or erythromycin. Occasionally long-term antibiotic prophylaxis may be helpful in those patients who suffer frequent severe exacerbations through the winter months. It does not reduce the incidence of infection but probably diminishes the duration and severity of attacks. Bronchodilators are useful for some patients and occasional patients may benefit from corticosteroids. There is no sure way of predicting those who will benefit, short of a therapeutic trial, although the presence of wheezing and blood or sputum eosinophilia are useful pointers.

Sputum retention is a major problem in these patients. They should be encouraged to take fluids and shown how to do postural drainage where appropriate. Old-fashioned remedies such as steam inhalation can be soothing. Mucolytic drugs are virtually useless.

A common complaint in the elderly bronchitic is of troublesome cough at night. Codeine linctus (5 ml) in hot water can be most effective (Hughes, 1978). Graduated physical exercise can be most helpful in improving the exercise tolerance of the more severely disabled (Sinclair and Ingram, 1980).

Cor pulmonale is a not-uncommon terminal event in these patients. There is hypoxia with hypercapnoea, which may eventually lead to polycythaemia. The treatment is based on:

(1) rest and the prompt treatment of infection;
(2) diuretics;
(3) controlled oxygen therapy—some patients derive considerable benefit from domicillary oxygen therapy and oxygen walking aids;
(4) digoxin is not particularly helpful unless there is an actual arrhythmia (Doherty *et al.*, 1977);
(5) venesection;
(6) avoidance of sedatives.

RESPIRATORY FAILURE

Respiratory failure is of two distinct types:

(1) Hypoxaemia without carbon dioxide retention (e.g. asthma, pulmonary oedema, pulmonary emboli, etc.). The treatment is that of the underlying condition plus oxygen at 8 l/min by polymask or MC mask. Blood-gas estimations are necessary to monitor therapy.

(2) Hypoxaemia with carbon dioxide retention (e.g. chronic bronchitis/
   emphysema, severe status asthmaticus, drug overdosage, etc.).

Cyanosis is a diagnostic feature loved by medical tutors. However, it is
often not obviously present until P_aO_2 is below 50 mm Hg (6.7 kPa).
Blood-gas estimations are essential for proper assessment. The other
classical features of flapping tremor, twitching, and papilloedema do not
appear until there is gross elevation of the P_aCO_2. The aims of treatment
are to:

(1) improve alveolar ventilation;
(2) treat infection;
(3) remove excessive secretions.

Oxygen therapy MUST BE CONTROLLED CAREFULLY as the P_aO_2 may
rise sharply. The lower the P_aO_2 at the start of treatment, the more
sharply the P_aO_2 is likely to rise. It is essential that a mask designed to give
a controlled oxygen enrichment, e.g. 24%, 28% or 35%, be used, and
frequent blood-gas estimations and close observation of the patient's
clinical condition (especially drowsiness) be made. The oxygen therapy
must be continuous as intermittent therapy may provoke dangerously
large P_aO_2 variations.

In some patients respiratory stimulants may be useful as a short-term
measure. Their therapeutic and toxic levels are close and they must be
administered with caution. It is the authors' preference to use a doxap-
ram infusion as toxicity problems are considerably less common (see
Table 9.4).

The last resort is assisted ventilation. Careful selection of patients is
mandatory. The quality of life prior to the present episode must be
reasonable. There is little point in putting a severe respiratory cripple in

Table 9.4   Respiratory stimulant drugs

Drug	Dose	Side-effects
Doxapram	1–4 mg/min by infusion	Restlessness, vomiting Warmth and flushing during infusion Very occasionally convulsions
Nikethamide	0.5–2 g by slow in-jection ½-hourly	As above More prone to convulsions

Notes:
(1) These drugs must be used under careful supervision.
(2) Active physiotherapy is essential.

Table 9.5   Drug problems in patients with respiratory disease

(A) Exacerbation of existing respiratory disease by drugs
      (1) β-blockers   ⎫ Bronchoconstriction,
      (2) Aspirin   ⎬ especially in atopics
      (3) Cholinergic drugs, especially carbachol   ⎭ and asthmatics
      (4) Cholinergic drugs, especially carbachol   Increased bronchial
                                                                       secretions

(B) Altered drug sensitivity caused by respiratory disease
      (1) Increased sensitivity to digitalis
            (a) toxicity at lower digoxin levels (Hargreave, 1965; Paciaroni *et al.*, 1974);
            (b) altered digoxin distribution volume and clearance (Doherty *et al.*, 1977; du Souich *et al.*, 1978)
      (2) Possible induced metabolism of corticosteroids—due to increased hepatic microsomal enzyme activity (Dwyer *et al.*, 1967)
      (3) Reduced theophylline clearance in severe chronic obstructive airways disease and in heart failure (du Souich *et al.*, 1978; Ogilvie *et al.*, 1978)

a terminal illness on a ventilator, as it will be virtually impossible to wean him off again.

The treatment of pneumonia is outlined in Chapter 5.

PULMONARY TUBERCULOSIS

The incidence of this disease is declining more slowly in the elderly than in any other age group. Diagnosis in the aged may be hindered by atypical presentation. Even in post-primary tuberculosis the main symptoms may be non-specific (malaise and weight loss), with less prominent respiratory symptoms. In 'cryptic' miliary tuberculosis the diagnosis may only be made by liver biopsy or bone marrow culture, with no respiratory features present. Although these atypical presentations are commoner in the elderly, the majority of patients in this age group still present with typical symptoms. Tuberculin tests are often negative in the aged tuberculosis patient.

The standard regimen for pulmonary tuberculosis is not affected by age: isoniazid metabolism is not affected by age (Farah *et al.*, 1977) and no obvious age-related changes have been noted in either rifampicin or ethambutol pharmacokinetics. The standard regimen is isoniazid 300 mg and rifampicin 600 mg (450 mg if less than 50 kg) once daily for 9 months, supplemented by ethambutol 15 mg/kg for the first 2 months. In severe cases and in miliary tuberculosis the most bactericidal regimen available should be used: streptomycin 0.75–1 g i.m. daily, pyrazinamide

2.0 g (1.5 g if less than 50 kg) once daily and the above doses of rifampicin and isoniazid. The critically ill patient may also require steroids initially. All antituberculosis therapy should be supervised by a chest physician.

There are also problems relating to the use of drugs in the presence of respiratory disease. These problems are summarized in Table 9.5. Drugs may also produce lung problems. This aspect of iatrogenic disease is detailed in Table 9.6.

Table 9.6   Drugs producing respiratory symptoms

Pulmonary reaction	Drug
Allergic alveolitis/fibrosis	Busulphan
	Bleomycin
	Other cytotoxic drugs
	Ganglion-blockers (hexamethonium)
	Gold
	Methysergide
	Nitrofurantoin
Asthma	Aspirin
	Indomethacin
	Non-steroidal anti-inflammatory drugs
	β-blockers
	Prostaglandins
	MAOIs
	Iodides
	Iron dextran
Generalized reactions	INAH
	Gold
	Phenylbutazone
	Hydrallazine
	Methyldopa
	Phenytoin
Pulmonary eosinophilia	Nitrofurantoin
	PAS

Note:
Adverse pulmonary reactions to drugs are relatively uncommon. They may require corticosteroids. Usually but not always resolution occurs on removal of the drug.

182

REFERENCES AND BIBLIOGRAPHY

Davies, P. D. B. (1969) Drug-induced lung disease. *Brit. J. Dis. Chest*, **63**, 57.

Davies, P. (1976) Drug-induced lung disease. *Medicine (London)*, **22**, 1074.

Doherty, J. E. *et al.* (1977) Digitalis in pulmonary heart disease (cor pulmonale). *Drugs*, **13**, 142.

Du Souich, P. *et al.* (1978) Pulmonary disease and drug kinetics. *Clin. Pharmacokinet.*, **3**, 257.

Dwyer, J. *et al.* (1967) A study of cortisol metabolism in patients with chronic asthma. *Austr. Ann. Intern. Med.*, **16**, 297.

Farah, F., *et al.* (1977) Hepatic drug acetylation and oxidation: effects of ageing in man. *Brit. Med. J.*, **2**, 155–6.

Hargreave, F. E. (1965) Digitalis and cor pulmonale. *Brit. Med. J.*, **2**, 943.

Hughes, D. (1976) Chemoprophylaxis in chronic bronchitis. *J. Antimicrob. Ther.*, **2**, 320.

Hughes, D. T. D. (1978) Cough suppressants, expectorants and mucolytics. *Brit. Med. J.*, **1**, 1202.

Jusko, W. J. *et al.* (1977) Intravenous theophylline: nomogram guidelines. *Ann. Intern. Med.*, **86**, 400–04.

Macdonald, J. B. *et al.* (1976) Asthma deaths in Cardiff 1963–74: 53 deaths in hospital. *Brit. Med. J.*, **2**, 721–3.

McDevitt, D. G. (1978) β-adrenoreceptor antagonists and respiratory function. *Brit. J. Clin. Pharmacol.*, **4**, 491.

Murray, J. F. (1976) *The Normal Lung*. W. B. Saunders. Philadelphia, London, Toronto.

Ogilvie, R. I. (1978) Clinical pharmacokinetics of theophylline. *Clin. Pharmacokinet.*, **3**, 267.

Paciaroni, E. *et al.* (1974) Le digoxinemia nei soggetti con cuore pulmonare cronico. *Giomarle Gerontologi*, **22**, 832.

Peach, H. and Pathy, M. S. (1981) Follow-up study of disability among elderly patients discharged from hospital with exacerbations of chronic bronchitis. *Thorax*, **36**, 585–9.

Piafsky, K. M. *et al.* (1977a) Theophylline kinetics in patients with acute pulmonary oedema. *Clin. Pharmacol. Ther.*, **21**, 310–16.

Piafsky, K. M. *et al.* (1977b) Theophylline distribution in patients with hepatic cirrhosis. *New Engl. J. Med.*, **296**, 1495–7.

Powell, J. R. *et al.* (1978) Theophylline disposition in acutely ill hospitalised patients. *Am. Rev. Resp. Dis.*, **11**, 229–37.

Sinclair, D. J. M. and Ingram, C. G. (1980) Controlled trial of supervised exercise training in chronic bronchitis. *Brit. Med. J.*, **1**, 519–21.

Skinner, C. *et al.* (1975) Comparison of the effects of acetabulol and practolol on airways obstruction in asthmatics. *Brit. J. Clin. Pharmacol.*, **2**, 417.

Tuttle, C. B. and Sidorov, J. (1977) Correct use of aerosol inhalers. *Can. Med. Assoc. J.*, **117**, 21.

Chapter 10

Renal disease

In the elderly the main problems affecting the urinary tract are urinary tract infection, prostatic disease, renal failure, and, above all else, incontinence. Many other afflictions common in younger age groups are rare in the elderly and have therefore been omitted.

The main anatomical and physiological changes associated with advancing age have been summarized in Chapter 1.

URINARY TRACT INFECTION

Kunin (1974) found little evidence that recurrent urinary tract infections do serious renal damage in normal kidneys with normal urine flow. Where there are structural abnormalities the position is more serious. It is essential in all cases of urinary tract infection that the causative organism is identified. This is done by collecting a mid-stream specimen (or catheter specimen) of urine and submitting this to culture. The most common organisms are *E. coli* and *Proteus*. On giving the appropriate antibiotic, patients should be advised that symptomatic improvement will occur promptly but that it is important that the antibiotic course be completed. A high fluid intake is also beneficial. An early relapse is most likely to be due to a failure of patient compliance or an inadequate regimen (Daschner and Marget, 1975)

Long-term suppressive antibacterial therapy is usually only required where there is an irremediable structural abnormality or where it is impossible to eradicate the infection.

Men are troubled much less frequently than women by urinary tract infections. Male infections are frequently associated with prostatic disease, either prostatic enlargement or prostatitis. Where prostatitis is present it is best to use a basic drug such as cotrimoxazole or erythromycin which distribute well into the highly acidic prostatic fluid.

Renal tuberculosis is not unknown in the elderly. It may present as sterile pyuria, which should in all cases be followed by 3 EMU specimens for culture. The regimen at present used is:

> rifampicin 450 mg daily (600 mg if over 50 kg);
> isoniazid 300 mg daily;
> ethambutol 15 mg/kg daily for the first 2 months.

At present there is no clear evidence as to how long therapy should be continued. Nine months' therapy is regarded as the minimum and many physicians prefer 18 months' chemotherapy. Unfortunately, ureteric stenosis is a common complication of renal tuberculosis. Corticosteroids (prednisolone 20 mg daily) have been advocated to prevent this occurring, but their efficacy is disputed.

PROSTATIC DISEASE

Some degree of prostatic enlargement occurs in virtually all men with advancing years. The main approach in severe cases is surgical, with medical therapy being confined to the treatment of infection.

Carcinoma of the prostate is also relatively common in elderly men. Stilboestrol is extremely effective in shrinking the carcinoma and may diminish metastases. The doses recommended vary enormously from 1 mg to 500 mg daily. Most physicians would use 1–3 mg daily. The best guide is the response of the individual patient. Other possible therapies in carcinoma of the prostate are radiotherapy or castration.

CHRONIC RENAL FAILURE

If possible try to establish if there is any underlying cause which may be treated. Usually no specific therapy is possible and medical care is directed at preserving what function is left in the compromised kidneys (Curtis and Williams, 1975). The therapeutic approaches to this problem are outlined in Table 10.1.

It is also essential to remember that drugs may precipitate renal problems (Table 10.2) and that renal impairment is one of the greatest influences on the handling of drugs, e.g. digoxin (see Table 10.3). The incidence of adverse drug reactions increases in renal impairment (Smith *et al.*, 1966; Jick, 1977). The response to a drug may be enhanced with the accumulation of active metabolites (Drayer, 1976).

Table 10.1   Medical management of chronic renal failure

(A) *Water*	Impairment of concentrating power	Risk of hyponatraemia and water intoxication
	Ability to form free water decreased	
	Treat by: water restriction—assess for each individual patient	
(B) *Sodium*	Obligatory loss increases (may develop a salt-losing state)	
	Treat by: careful individual monitoring of serum sodium and urinary sodium loss	

<table>
<tr><td>(C) Potassium</td><td>Potassium excretion is usually well maintained. Avoid drugs which increase potassium load, e.g. spironolactone
Treat hyperkalaemia: emergency but temporary therapy is:
(a) calcium gluconate 1 mg in 10 ml; if acidotic—isotonic sodium bicarbonate
(b) 10 units insulin with 25 g glucose
(c) ion exchange resins
(d) peritoneal/haemodialysis</td></tr>
<tr><td>(D) Acidosis</td><td>Treat acidosis when venous bicarbonate >20 mmol/l by giving sodium bicarbonate. Dose must be individually adjusted.</td></tr>
<tr><td>(E) Uraemia</td><td>Treat by: 20 g first-class protein diet with 2000 cal from carbohydrate and fat
Intermittent haemodialysis when on 30–40 g protein diet does not keep the blood urea below 200 mg/100 ml (35 mmol/l)</td></tr>
<tr><td>(F) Anaemia</td><td>Iron is sometimes beneficial; try to avoid transfusions.</td></tr>
</table>

Table 10.2   Drugs causing renal impairment

(1) Acute tubular necrosis	Penicillins Aminoglycosides Gold and other heavy metals Solvents, e.g. carbon tetrachloride Salicylates Cephaloridine Lithium
(2) Acute interstitial nephritis/arteritis Via direct toxic effect, and by immune complex damage	Anticonvulsants Penicillins Sulphonamides Thiazides Anticoagulants Rifampicin Gold and penicillamine
(3) SLE syndrome	Hydralazine Procainamide Isoniazid, PAS, streptomycin Methyldopa Phenytoin Reserpine
(4) Drug-induced nephrotic syndrome	Gold Anticonvulsants Hypoglycaemics

Table 10.2   continued

(5) Analgesic nephropathy	Phenacetin/aspirin
(6) Uraemia by interfering with protein metabolism	Tetracycline/oxytetracycline, especially in the elderly Steroids
(7) Retroperitoneal fibrosis	Methysergide Hydralazine Diuretics Methyldopa
(8) Drugs producing metabolic changes (a) Hypokalaemia	Laxative abuse Diuretics Carbenoxolone Corticosteroids
Reduces renal concentrating ability Predisposes to infection May result in nephrogenic diabetes insipidus	
(a) Hypercalcaemia	Milk–alkali syndrome Steroids Vitamin D Acetazolamide
(c) Hyperuricaemia	Thiazide diuretics Cytotoxics
(9) Blood volume changes (a) Hypovolaemia	Tetracycline Ampicillin } Particularly likely in the elderly Diuretics
(b) Hypervolaemia	Ampicillin Carbenicillin Erythromycin

Table 10.3   Influence of renal impairment on drug handling

Drug	Effect of renal impairment	Clinical manifestation	Dosage in severe renal impairment	Reference
Penicillin	Plasma half-life increased	Encephalo-pathy in high dose	As normal	Conway *et al*, 1968
	Electrolyte imbalance	Hypokalaemia/ hyperkalaemia		Klastersky *et al.*, 1973 Tullet, 1970

Drug				Reference
Carbenicillin	Electrolyte imbalance	Hypokalaemia and alkalosis Convulsions Bleeding tendency	1 g/12–16 h	Hoffman *et al.*, 1970 Waisbren *et al.*, 1971
Cephalothin	Prolonged half-life	Convulsions Haemolytic anaemia	500 mg/8–12 h	Wu *et al.*, 1978
Gentamicin	Prolonged half-life	Ototoxicity Blockade of neuro-muscular transmission Nephrotoxicity	80 mg/24–48 h (control by trough levels)	Jackson and Arcieri, 1971 Appel and Neu, 1978
Cotrimoxa-zole	Reduced excretion		One tablet twice daily where creatinine clearance less than 15 ml/min	Hansen, 1978
Tetracyclines*	Avoid even where mild renal impairment			
Digoxin	Prolonged half-life due to decreased excretion	Digoxin toxicity	Monitor levels; reduce dose and/or increase dosage interval	Gault *et al.*, 1976
β-adreno-receptor blocking agents	Metabolism reduced Excretion of metabolites reduced		Reduce dosage	
Potassium-sparing diuretics	Produce hyperkalaemia		Avoid	
Thiazide diuretics	Accumulate	Ototoxicity	Avoid	
Chloroprop-amide	Prolonged half-life Accumulation of metabolites	Hypoglycaemia	Reduce dose	Fabre and Balant, 1976

Table 10.3 continued

Drug	Effect of renal impairment	Clinical manifestation	Dosage in severe renal impairment	Reference
Phenytoin	Less bound to plasma protein More rapidly metabolized		Use normal dose	Odar-Cederloff and Borga, 1974
Cimetidine	Excretion delayed	Confusion Convulsions	Reduce dose	Schentag *et al.*, 1979

INCONTINENCE

This problem is widespread and demoralizing in the extreme. Over 2 million people in the United Kingdom are estimated to be incontinent (Editorial, 1978). Many suffer in silence, ashamed to ask for help. All too often when they do seek help they are met with indifference. Although present in 7.6% of men and 12.5% of women over 65 years, the problem is not confined to the elderly. It has been estimated that in the age range 1–64 years about 2% of men and 7.5% of women are incontinent.

For many women the problem of stress incontinence dates back to childbirth in earlier life. Accurate assessment is required as in the main the treatment is surgical (Editorial, 1977). In elderly women suffering from senile vaginitis urinary incontinence can be an associated problem. This is due to the close relationship of the trigone of the bladder and the vagina. The oestrogen therapy used for the vaginitis may also relieve the incontinence.

Fortunately much incontinence is temporary, due to immobility and illness. It disappears when the patient recovers. If catheterization is required it should be done for the shortest possible time. A thorough aseptic technique should be used for insertion.

Overflow incontinence can be due to urinary retention. In men this may be secondary to prostatic enlargement. However, in both sexes probably the most common cause of this type of incontinence is constipation. The incontinence disappears with proper attention to the bowel problem.

It is unfortunately common for urge incontinence to be associated with strokes and dementia. This is due to reduction or loss of the power to inhibit micturition.

The attitudes of the people caring for the elderly also play a part in the incidence of incontinence. In those hospitals and homes operating enlightened policies, treating their elderly patients as human beings, the incidence of incontinence is reduced (DHSS, 1977). It is really basic common sense that those people who have a precarious control over their bladder function should have a bedside commode at night and that in the daytime they have a short distance, and easy access, to toilets.

There are several aspects of the promotion of continence, including drugs and habit. For those unfortunates who do not regain full continence a variety of aids exist.

In the promotion of continence regular visits to the toilet play an important part. This helps to establish a regular pattern of bladder-emptying. Rowe (1977) found a discreet light alarm reminder to be a useful adjunct to regular toilet training.

Several drugs are used in the treatment of incontinence. These are detailed in Table 10.4. The recent report on the effect of flunarizine (Palmer *et al.*, 1981) has been most encouraging. It was used to great effect in women with proven detrussor instability. No serious side-effects were encountered. It also has the great advantage of once-daily administration.

Emepromium bromide has been shown to be effective when administered intramuscularly (Brocklehurst *et al.*, 1972; Ritch *et al.*, 1977a,b). Its efficacy after oral administration is less certain (Ekeland and Sander,

Table 10.4   Drugs used in the treatment of urinary incontinence

Drug	Dosage	Side-effects	Contra-indications
Emepromium bromide	200 mg thrice daily If nocturnal fre- frequency 200–400 mg nocte with water	Oesophageal ulceration Anticholinergic effects	Glaucoma Oesophagitis
Flavoxate hydro-chloride	200 mg thrice daily	As above	As above
Flunarizine	200 mg nocte	Drowsiness Increased perspira- tion Hypotonic bladder Peripheral oedema	

1976; Ritch *et al.*, 1977a,b). The effectiveness of flavoxate (Stanton, 1973) is equally uncertain.

Where it is not possible to restore continence fully it is still worth while trying to reduce incontinence to a minimum. In these cases external appliances will be required. Penile clamps and the female equivalent belong in the dark ages. In the male patient a condom urinal may well be successful. It does, however, require a great degree of patient co-operation. For both men and women the marsupial pants (Dr F. L. Willington) are a great boon. They are made of one-way water-repellent material with a pad on the outside in a waterproof pouch. The pads can be changed without removing the pants. It is vital that the pants fit as snugly as possible.

Where incontinence pads/napkins are used in bed it is essential that they are positioned properly, with the bonded end across the bed.

For some patients long-term catheterization will still be required. This is not a decision to be taken lightly. Carefully and delicate enquiry may need to be made to discover if the couple are still sexually active. Great care must be taken to preserve the dignity of the patient. Nobody wants to walk around carrying a urinary drainage bag. Leg bags can be discreetly attached under skirts or trousers, and provided a flutter valve is used reflux is not a problem. It is also possible to affix the bag round the patient's waist (Shepheard's Sporran). The newer catheters are much less irritant and can last 2 months between changes. All long-term catheter patients have infected urine. Long-term continuous medication makes not one whit of difference; indeed in the elderly in hot weather it can be positively disadvantageous (Macdonald and Macdonald, 1976). Short courses of antibiotics are necessary if the patient has symptoms of a urinary tract infection.

Where elderly incontinence patients are being managed at home, it is essential that the families be given the maximum amount of support and help (e.g. supply of pads, local authority washing service, etc.). Occasional admissions to hospital for family relief may enable the patient to be maintained at home for much longer than might otherwise be possible.

REFERENCES AND BIBLIOGRAPHY

Appel, G. B. and Neu, H. C. (1978) Nephrotoxicity of antimicrobial agents. *New Engl. J. Med.*, **296**, 663.

Brocklehurst, J. C. *et al.* (1972) Emepromium bromide in urinary incontinence. *Age and Ageing*, **1**, 152–7.

Cardozo, L. D. *et al.* (1980) Evaluation of fluribprofen in detrusor instability. *Brit. Med. J.*, **280**, 281–2.

Conway, N. *et al.* (1968) Penicillin encephalopathy. *Postgrad. Med. J.*, **44**, 891.

Curtis, J. R. and Williams, G. B. (1975) *Clinical Management of Chronic Renal Failure.* Blackwell, Oxford.

Daschner, F. and Marget, W. (1975) Treatment of recurrent urinary tract infection in children: compliance with regimen. *Acta Paediat. Scand.*, **64**, 105.

DHSS (1977) *Residential Homes for the Elderly: Arrangements for Health Care.* HMSO, London.

Drayer, D. E. (1976) Pharmacologically active metabolites. *Clin. Pharmacokinet.*, **1**, 426.

Editorial (1977) Stress incontinence. *Brit. Med. J.*, **2**, 2.

Editorial (1978) Incontinence. *Brit. Med. J.*, **1**, 61–2.

Ekeland, A. and Sander, S. (1976) A urodynamic study of emepromium bromide in bladder dysfunction. *Scand. J. Urol. Nephrol.*, **10**, 195.

Fabre, J. and Balant, L. (1976) Renal failure, drug pharmacokinetics and drug action. *Clin. Pharmacokinet.*, **1**, 99.

Frewen, W. K. (1980) The management of urgency and frequency of micturition. *Br. J. Urol.*, **52**, 367–9.

Gault, M. H. *et al.* (1976) Studies of digoxin dosage, kinetics and serum concentrations in renal failure. *Nephron*, **17**, 161.

Hansen, I. B. (1978) The combination of trimethoprim–sulphamethoxazole. In . Schonfeld (ed.), *Antibiotics and Chemotherapy*, vol. 25, p. 217. Karger, Basel.

Hoffman, T. A. *et al.* (1970) Pharmacodynamics of carbenicillin in hepatic and renal failure. *Ann. Intern. Med.*, **73**, 173.

Jackson, C. G. and Arcieri, G. (1971) Ototoxicity of gentamicin in man. *J. Infect. Dis.*, **124** (suppl.), S130.

Jick, H. (1977) Adverse drug effects in relation to renal function. *Am. J. Med.*, **62**, 514.

Klastersky, J. *et al.* (1973) Carbenicillin and hypokalaemia. *Ann. Intern. Med.*, **78**, 774.

Kunin, C. N. (1974) *Detection, Prevention and Management of Urinary Tract Infection.* Lea & Febiger, Philadelphia.

Macdonald, J. B. and Macdonald, E. T. (1976) Nitrofurantoin crystalluria. *Brit. Med. J.*, **2**, 1004–5.

Odar-Cederloff, I. and Borga, O. (1974) Kinetics of diphenylhydantoin in uraemic patients. *Eur. J. Clin. Pharmacol.*, **7**, 31.

Palmer, J. H. *et al.* (1981) Flunarizine: a once-daily therapy for urinary incontinence. *Lancet*, **2**, 279–81.

Ritch, A. E. S. *et al.* (1977a) Emepromium bromide in urinary incontinence. *Lancet*, **1**, 799.

Ritch, A. E. S. *et al.* (1977b) Second look at emepromium bromide in urinary incontinence. *Lancet*, **1**, 504–6.

Rowe, P. S. (1977) Incontinence in the elderly. *Age and Ageing*, **6**, 238.

Rud, T. *et al.* (1979) Effects of calcium antagonists in women with unstable bladders. *Urol. Int.*, **34**, 421–9.

Schentag, J. J. *et al.* (1979) Pharmacokinetic and clinical studies with cimetidine associated mental confusion. *Lancet*, **1**, 177.

Smith, J. W. *et al.* (1966) Studies on the epidemiology of adverse drug reactions. V. Clinical factors influencing susceptibility. *Ann. Intern. Med.*, **65**, 629.

Stanton, S. L. (1973) A comparison of emepromium bromide and flavoxate hydrochloride in the treatment of urinary incontinence. *J. Urol.*, **110**, 529–32.

Thomas, T. M. *et al.* (1980) The prevalence of incontinence in the community. *Brit. Med. J.*, **281**, 1243.

Tullet, G. L. (1970) Sudden death occurring during 'massive-dose' potassium penicillin G. therapy. *Wisc. Med. J.*, **69**, 216.

Waisbren, B. A. *et al.* (1971) Carbenicillin and bleeding. *JAMA*, **217**, 1243.

Wu, M. J. *et al.* (1978) Cephalothin neurotoxicity in renal failure. *Ann. Intern. Med.*, **89**, 429.

Section Three

Chapter 11

Background to patient compliance

Compliance has been defined as the extent to which a person's behaviour (in terms of taking medication, etc.) coincides with medical advice (Haynes *et al.*, 1979). This wide-ranging definition would include events which neither the doctor nor the patient can influence, such as a pharmacist altering a precription or giving the medication in an unsuitable container. We feel that the above definition is casting the net too wide, and would restrict the term compliance to all the events between the consultation and the ingestion of the medication over which the patient has control. We feel this is what the term means to most doctors. The restriction is intended merely to identify which links in the chain of events are being discussed, and does not imply that the patient is the root of all compliance problems. In fact, compliance is strongly affected by many aspects of the treatment system (not least, doctors) as we shall discuss later.

Compliance has two aspects. To comply, the patient must firstly be mentally able to take the regimen if he or she so wishes. This implies that he first comprehends the regimen; then has the mental capacity to integrate the regimen into his daily life; and is not prevented from taking his drugs by mental factors such as loss of memory, disorientation, or psychiatric disease. Secondly, he must wish to take his drugs. This wish must be strong enough to motivate him to remember and to take his drugs at the correct time. This wish will be influenced by a host of background factors. Compliance is a lot wider and deeper than the patient just happening to forget to take the medication.

Several of the underwritten assumptions and attitudes lying behind compliance merit consideration before examining the phenomenon itself. Perhaps the most important is that many of the terms used carry definite moral overtones—'irregular', 'defaulter', 'unmotivated', 'lapsed patient', etc. As a leading article in *Tubercle* put it: 'the use of words implying moral judgements tends to clear the mind of doubt and to discourage curiosity about causes' (Leading article, 1970). Although happily this moralizing attitude is becoming less common, non-compliance still 'has about it a flavour of disobedience—behaviour unacceptable to a traditionally authoritarian profession' (Editorial, 1979).

But is this disciplinarian view fair or sensible? Vlasak (1969) has commented that treatment is nearly always viewed from the doctor's point of view. Until recently relatively little had been done to assess the patients' attitudes and opinions. Usually the central question is: how can we get the patient to comply? This 'management bias' has been a hardy tradition in medicine, both in clinical practice and medical research. It has been well described by Roth (1962). For instance, Levine *et al.* (1969) have commented that doctors or nurses are rarely considered to have any problems in their own attitude or behaviour which might impede doctor–patient understanding. The increasing importance being given to compliance suggests that medical insight is growing.

Nonetheless there are two points of view in the doctor–patient relationship. To understand compliance problems we must try to see the situation through the patients' eyes. Some studies (BTTA, 1971; Grzybowski *et al.*, 1965) have shown that a few non-compliant patients have overt psychiatric disease and doubtless other patients have minor psychiatric problems. However, many patients who stop taking their medication do so as a result of a decision that is for them both sensible and balanced. This decision is based on their knowledge of the disease and their experience of the treatment system (Rouillon, 1972). It balances the gains they expect from the therapy against the inconvenience of attending clinics, taking tablets, side-effects, and so on. Personal attitudes and personality also play a part. Rouillon (1972) has emphasized that non-compliance should be viewed first as a failure of the treatment system. The act of prescribing a drug is a direct statement from the doctor that the therapy is desirable and that benefits will outweigh the inconveniences. If the patient does not appreciate this, it indicates that the doctor has failed to explain to him in terms he can understand and with an approach he can accept. If the patient's decision is taken in ignorance of the basic facts then that is the physician's fault. Relatively few studies have examined patients' knowledge of their disease. Vandiviere (1970) studied the knowledge tuberculous patients have of their disease. Only half knew the disease was contagious and only 20% knew the names of all their drugs. Several other studies have been made, usually in the context of improving compliance by education. The results are difficult to assess but the overall picture is not reassuring.

The other factor is patient motivation. Rouillon (1969 and 1972) has made several perceptive analyses of motivation. She considers that the act of non-compliance is rarely an isolated event. A patient's behaviour is largely the result of a long chain of conscious or unconscious influences he has undergone within the treatment system. With preventive or long-term medication the treatment system has to sell the patient an idea that is clearly absurd on crude 'common-sense' grounds. That idea is that he should continue to take tablets, possibly with disagreeable taste or side-effects, long after he himself feels perfectly healthy. Prime examples of this are antihypertensives and antituberculous drugs. The patient is also required to take the therapy with more regularity and dedication than he applies to almost anything else he does not absolutely have to do. To persuade the patient to invest considerable effort into such a project he will have to be thoroughly convinced. Thus the doctor does not start on neutral ground; he starts with the odds already stacked against him. Unless the idea is put over to the patient very effectively, common sense is likely to win and the medication be stopped.

Rouillon (1969, 1972) has also pointed out several paradoxes in our current thinking on compliance. Firstly, it is beyond the power of human beings to be always regular and obedient. To err is human. To be prepared to go on for ever swallowing drugs each day without any reinforcement requires a coldly intellectual or an obsessive personality. Dedicated regularity is itself abnormal. Secondly, we ask each outpatient to play two incompatible roles simultaneously. He must play the role of the invalid faithfully obeying his doctor's orders; but at the same time he has to play the role of the healthy person—independent, making his own decisions, and going about his everyday life as usual. No wonder these roles sometimes clash. The third paradox is that any efficient treatment system produces standardization with its tendency to dehumanize and alienate. Only by fighting against this tendency can we gain and retain our patient's full co-operation.

One curious simile for compliance has been noted by Jonsen (1979): 'As I read through the literature on compliance, I am struck by how much it resembles, save for the statistics and controlled trials, the problems faced by the minister charged with leading his parishioners to the godly life.' He concludes that compliance poses much the same problems as piety: even the best intentions become quickly ensnared in the flaws of the human condition. The doctor has many similar problems to the priest. He knows The Truth: how can he best lead his wayward flock towards the light?

The term compliance is itself controversial. Several authors dislike its authoritarian overtones, and have suggested more neutral terms such as adherence. Society is today redefining the relationship between doctors and patients. We are evolving towards a more relaxed realistic system of equal partnership. The connotations of 'compliance' may seem to fly in the face of this evolution. It appears, however, that 'compliance' is accepted and here to stay.

In the last decade compliance has become academically respectable. It has entered the Hall of Fame and is listed in *Index Medicus* (as 'Patient Compliance', 'Patient Dropouts'). Ivan Illich has even added it to his long list of medical crimes. The most tangible evidence of interest is the number of papers published per year. By all these standards compliance has come of age.

MEASURING COMPLIANCE

The act of compliance is essentially private. Any attempt to measure it is an intrusion into this privacy which runs the risk of distorting the observed act. So compliance measurement is essentially indirect (apart from the rare cases where para-medical staff give out medication directly, e.g. depot phenothiazines). Methods of measuring compliance are shown in Table 11.1.

The most direct method of measuring compliance is to measure the drug's presence in the patient's blood or urine, or the presence in the urine of a metabolite or a marker drug given with it. In theory almost any drug or metabolite detectable in blood or urine could be used. Suitable detection methods are available for most antibiotics and antituberculosis drugs, phenothiazines, tricyclic antidepressants, nearly all antiepileptic drugs, benzodiazepines, digoxin, thiazides, β-blockers, methyldopa, non-steroidal anti-inflammatory drugs, and oral hypoglycaemics (Haynes *et al.*, 1979). Porter (1969) has given the requirements for an ideal urine marker drug (Table 11.2). Several suitable drugs are available. However, formulations containing marker drugs need to be specially prepared so are only useful in compliance research.

The major disadvantage of measuring drug levels is that they only measure compliance on the day of ingestion (or sometimes up to a maximum of 2 or 3 days). A patient could take his tablets only on clinic days and still register complete compliance. Testing at random home visits could detect this problem, but this requires time and personnel and is probably only feasible in the research setting. Two other problems can also occur with these techniques. Firstly, the detection methods must be reliable and not influenced by other drugs or food. Also the sample must be taken during the excretion period. For example, a late-afternoon clinic urine sample for rifampicin can be negative if the patient has taken his tablets as usual some 8–9 h before. The second problem is of between-individual variations in pharmacokinetics which can give widely varying serum levels for the same dose. This can sometimes make the lower limits for adequate compliance difficult to set: is the patient a poor complier or a rapid metabolizer? Despite their drawbacks, however, these biochemical methods are the only techniques which prove incontrovertibly that the patient has taken his tablets.

A variety of more indirect methods are available (see Table 11.1). Perhaps the most indirect method is to use the outcome of treatment as a measure of drug compliance. If the patient gets better he must be taking his tablets. Most doctors frequently use this train of thought, perhaps only subconsciously. Its many shortcomings are evident. It assumes that improvement can only be brought about by fully compliant treatment: spontaneous recovery does not occur and partial compliance gives no benefit. If one looks at a common clinical problem like the antibiotic therapy of acute bronchitis one sees the flaws in these assumptions.

Table 11.1   Methods for measuring compliance

Direct methods
(1) Blood levels of drug
(2) Urinary excretion of:
    (a) drug
    (b) metabolite
    (c) marker drug

Indirect methods
(1) Outcome of treatment
(2) Doctor's subjective opinion
(3) Direct patient questioning
(4) Pill counts
(5) Monitoring repeat prescriptions
(6) Medication monitors

Table 11.2   Requirements for an ideal urine tracer drug to assess compliance

(1) Non-toxic and pharmacologically inert
(2) Unaffected by urine variables (pH, temperature, other constituents)
(3) Rapidly and completely excreted in the urine (peak within 2–3 h of ingestion and undetectable after about 6 h)
(4) Non-cumulative
(5) Simple, quick, sensitive, and specific detection methods available.
(6) Not detectable in the urine from diet or self-medication sources
(7) Patient unable to detect the marker by colour, odour, etc.

Using therapeutic outcome also involves other less obvious assumptions. For instance, other aspects of medical care (reassurance, sympathy, etc.) should have no effect, and other medications (prescribed and patent) should have no effect on the outcome being examined. A further problem is that good treatment must always give success. In one study only 16% of patients on thiazides had controlled hypertension when they had negative urine tests, but 44% had controlled hypertension with positive urine tests. Thus compliance significantly reduced blood pressure. But the majority (56%) of compliers had uncontrolled blood pressure and would be deemed non-compliers if therapeutic outcome had been the sole criterion (Lowenthal *et al.*, 1976); so therapeutic outcome is fraught with dangers as an index of compliance. It is only valid when all the preconditions above have been fulfilled. Such occasions are rare.

The next most 'common-sense' method of assessing compliance is the doctor's assessment of the patient's ability to take the drugs regularly. But are doctors any good at this assessment? Mushlin and Appel (1977) investigated the ability of junior hospital doctors to predict whether inpatients would return for a follow-up appointment after discharge, or would take their digitalis and diuretics correctly. Their performance at identifying the non-attenders was bad but the prediction of those failing to take their therapy was awful. Caron and Roth (1968) found that housemen were unable to predict medical compliance with antacid regimens. The results were no better than you would expect by chance. Moulding (1970) compared physicians' predictions with records on a medication monitor (a neat device to record the time at which a patient dispenses his own medication). He found that, of patients predicted to have good (90%+) compliance, 20% had only moderate (70–90%) compliance and 6% had poor (below 70%) compliance. Conversely, of patients predicted to have poor compliance, 33% had moderate compliance. Doctors predicted 51% of the poor or moderate compliers. The relatively good predictive results in this study may reflect the fact that it used highly experienced doctors, interested in compliance. So this study may represent nearly the best that doctors can achieve, while the two previous studies may be nearer the norm. The overall conclusion must be that doctors predict patient compliance poorly.

One other simple way of measuring compliance is simply to ask the patient whether he is taking all his tablets. The sceptic might quote Socrates who stated that the doctor 'should remain aware of the fact that patients often lie when they say that they have taken certain medicines'. But recent studies comparing questioning with other techniques have provided some helpful and reassuring answers. The questioning must be performed in a neutral and non-aggressive manner such as: 'Most people forget to take their tablets sometimes. Do you find it difficult to remember?' Park and Lipman (1964) compared direct questioning with pill counts in 117 psychiatric outpatients. Of 100 patients stating that they were fully compliant, 39% were moderately non-compliant by pill counts (more than 66% of tablets taken) and 6% were markedly non-compliant. Of 9 patients reporting mild non-compliance, 6 indeed were mildly non-compliant and 1 markedly non-compliant. Of 8 reporting major non-compliance, 7 were telling the truth and 1 was only mildly non-compliant. Feinstein *et al.* (1959) also found excellent correlation between pill counts and interviews for non-compliance but a poorer correlation for good compliers. Sackett *et al.* (1976) conducted similar studies in hypertensives. This study found that 91% of patients admitting non-compliance were telling the truth. Several other smaller studies have produced similar results. While it is depressing to realize that substantial numbers of patients do not take their medication, it is important to remember that if patients admit they are not taking their tablets they are virtually always telling the truth. Some 50% of serious non-compliers admit this on questioning. There is also evidence that it is this group who admit their non-compliance who respond best to efforts to improve compliance. So direct questioning is simple, practical, and effective in everyday practice.

The major standard of comparison so far for other methods of measuring compliance has been the pill count. It compares the amount of medication remaining with the amount that should have been left, based on date of prescription and dose frequency. This is a popular method, but how good is it?

Bergman and Werner (1963) compared pill counts with urine tests in children receiving antibiotics. By day three 46% of patients were complying by urine tests and 44% by pill count. By day nine of the ten-day course 8% were complying by urine test and 18% by pill counts. So pill counts tended to over-estimate compliance. Roth *et al.* (1970) again found a tendency for pill counts to overestimate compliance.

Pill counts are best carried out at a surprise home visit. This is time-consuming and only feasible in a research setting. In clinical practice pill counts are really only possible in the surgery or outpatient clinic. Here they have substantial problems (see Table 11.3). These many problems severely limit the value of pill counting in everyday life. As a research tool it is probably less reliable than is often assumed.

Monitoring repeat prescriptions is essentially a large-scale version of pill counting. It compares the expected and actual frequency with which

Table 11.3   Problems with pill counts

---

(1) Limited access: poor compliers are the ones most likely to forget to bring their medication to the clinic for counting.
(2) Overtness: discreet pill counts are difficult to achieve: The sense of surveillance could improve compliance but may just encourage disposal of unconsumed tablets before the next visit.
(3) Lack of surprise: pill numbers can be 'adjusted' if counting is expected.
(4) Tablet-swapping: causes an overestimation of compliance. This is discussed later in the text.
(5) Use of old medication: many patients on chronic medication have small reserve stocks of old medication. If these are used compliance can be misleading.
(6) Timing of prescription: most patients renew their medication before the previous supply is exhausted. Thus pill counting from the bottle date can be misleading.

---

the patients repeat their prescriptions. Many general practitioners use this method to detect gross non-compliance. In our own locality tuberculosis health visitors monitor the repeat prescriptions to assess the compliance with the antituberculosis regimens. This is only feasible in a confined area and takes more time than would be available in normal circumstances. Routine monitoring of repeat prescriptions could be incorporated into the prescribing pattern in general practice surgeries. If the doctor were automatically alerted to overdue repeat medication, compliance could be substantially improved.

Monitoring repeat prescription and pill counting do not measure actual ingestion. That is still only an assumption. During a home visit for a compliance study in Nottingham we found that an old lady had conscientiously repeated her hypnotic prescription every 2 months for 10 years. Although she never took the tablets, she felt she might offend her doctor by failing to repeat her prescription. She kept the unused tablets in the bottom drawer of her wardrobe. While this must be an extreme case, more minor degrees of tablet hoarding seem fairly common and are not detected by prescription monitoring.

A medication monitor is a drug dispenser with a time recording device for determining when patients remove medication. Potentially it could offer the most accurate means of all of assessing compliance. Its only potential disadvantage is again that removal need not equate with ingestion. However, errors of this type are more detectable: to fool the monitor the patient needs to remove his medication regularly every day. Such dedication and regularity are uncommon among non-compliant patients. Several types of medication monitor have been described

(Moulding, 1979). The original device was described by Moulding (1967)—a device similar to a small confectionery vending machine. As each tray is removed, the stack drops down. A small piece of radioactive uranium is attached to the top of the stack and a strip of photographic or X-ray paper runs down the side of the dispenser. The uranium radiation creates a series of dots on the film. The size of the dot shows how long has elapsed between tray removals and the distance between dots shows if more than one tray has been removed at once. So far this has only been used as a research tool and its large potential has not yet been realized.

Hahn and Yee (1974) have developed an electronic device for similar measurements, but at present this is not widely used.

The medication monitor is by far the best method for studying drug removal in detail. Used in conjunction with blood or urine analysis at surprise visits, a rigorous analysis of compliance can be achieved. This combination should be the standard against which other measuring techniques should be gauged.

The one sizeable medication monitor trial (Moulding *et al.*, 1970) showed a good corelation between monitor and urine tests. It also displayed that there is a sizeable variation in compliance from day to day. This important fact, that compliance varies with time, has implications which vary with the particular therapy being used. For example, 50% compliance with a once-daily regimen could mean alternate-day medication (adequate for antituberculosis regimens or steroids but not for antihypertensive therapy) (Macdonald, 1979) or alternating weeks of 100% and 0% compliance (virtually always unsatisfactory). Thus the average compliance over several weeks is an approximation which may hide a range of clinical effectiveness behind one figure.

It is plain that compliance is a much more complex concept than it appears at first sight. It is also inherently difficult to study. Luckily, the intellectual rigour the subject demands is increasingly being seen as a challenge by able researchers. The quality of published studies is rising rapidly. We shall look at the results obtained so far in the following chapters.

REFERENCES AND BIBLIOGRAPHY

Bergman, A. B. and Werner, R. J. (1963) Failure of children to receive penicillin by mouth. *New Engl. J. Med.*, **268**, 1334–8.
BTTA (British Thoracic and Tuberculosis Association) (1971) A survey of tuberculosis mortality in England and Wales in 1968. *Tubercle*, **52**, 1.
Caron, H. S. and Roth, H. P. (1968) Patients' co-operation with a medical regimen. *JAMA*, **203**, 922–6.

Editorial (1979) Non-compliance—does it really matter? *Brit. Med. J.*, **2**, 1168.

Feinstein, A. R. *et al.* (1959) Streptococcal prophylaxis. *N. Engl. J. Med.*, **260**, 697–702.

Grzybowski, S. *et al.* (1965) Reactivations in pulmonary tuberculosis. *Am. Rev. Resp. Dis.*, **93**, 352.

Haynes, R. B., Taylor, D. W., and Sackett, D. L. (eds) (1979), *Compliance in Health Care*. Johns Hopkins University Press, Baltimore.

Jonsen, A. R. (1979) Ethical issues. In R. B. Haynes *et al.* (eds), *Compliance in Health Care*, p. 113. Johns Hopkins University Press, Baltimore.

Leading article (1970) Supervision and defaulting. *Tubercle*, **51**, 100.

Levine, J. *et al.* (1969) Unravelling technology and culture in public health. *Am. J. Pub. Health*, **59**, 237.

Lowenthal, D. T. *et al.* (1976) Patient compliance for antihypertensive medication: the usefulness of urine assays. *Curr. Ther. Res.*, **19**, 405–9.

Macdonald, J. B. (1979) The origin of treatment failure in tuberculosis. M.D. Thesis, University of Cambridge.

Moulding, T. S. (1967) Vertical pill calendar dispenser for improving self-medication. *Tubercle*, **48**, 32–7.

Moulding, T. S. *et al.* (1970) Supervision of outpatient drug therapy with a medication monitor. *Arch. Intern. Med.*, **73**, 559.

Moulding, T. S. *et al.* (1979) The unrealised potential of the medication monitor. *Clin. Pharmacol. Ther.*, **25**, 131–6.

Mushlin, A. I. and Appel, F. A. (1977) Diagnosing patient non-compliance. *Arch. Intern. Med.*, **137**, 318–21.

Park, L. C. and Lipman, R. S. (1964) A comparison of patient dosage deviation reports with pill counts. *Psychopharmacologia*, **6**, 299–302.

Porter, A. M. (1969) Drug defaulting in general practice. *Brit. Med. J.*, **1**, 218.

Roth, J. A. (1962) 'Management bias' in social science study of medical treatment. *Hum. Org.*, **21**, 47.

Roth, H. P. *et al.* (1970) Measuring intake of medication: bottle count v. tracer technique. *Clin. Pharmacol. Ther.*, **11**, 228–37.

Rouillon, A. (1969) How to motivate patients to understand and pursue their treatment. *Bull. Int. Union Tuberc.*, **42**, 155.

Rouillon, A. (1972) What is motivation? *Bull. Int. Union Tuberc.*, **47**, 69.

Sackett, D. L. *et al.* (1976) The problem of compliance with antihypertensive therapy. *Pract. Cardiol.*, **2**, 35–9.

Vandiviere, H. M. (1970) The tuberculous patient's knowledge about his disease. *Am. Rev. Resp. Dis.*, **101**, 314.

Vlasak, G. J. (1969) A few characteristics of patients in urban tuberculosis clinics. *Publ. Health Rep.*, **84**, 159.

Yee, R. D. *et al.* (1974) Medication monitor for ophthalmology. *Am. J. Ophthalmol.*, **78**, 774–8.

Chapter 12

Problems of prescriptions and packets

BETWEEN PRESCRIPTION AND INGESTION

Every year drug companies spend many millions of pounds on developing new drugs to the point where they are testable on humans. Then clinical researchers expend a massive effort to assess each new drug's role. Original and review articles are written. Advertisements proliferate in the medical press. This whole process is now so complex, and the effort so huge, that the overall cost of marketing a new drug is now some £30 million. All these rapidly rising costs must eventually be paid for by the consumer.

Millions of pounds are thus spent before that magic moment when a doctor puts pen to prescription pad and prescribes a drug. But what happens after that moment? How much thought goes into ensuring that in real life drugs actually do the job they were tested for? This section will concentrate on what happens after the prescription is written. It will explore the still pitifully small effort that goes into assessing and improving the efficacy of prescribing.

In the past this area has received scant attention, although compliance is now becoming an acceptable area for research. Several reasons lie behind this past neglect. Perhaps the most powerful has been a reluctance among individual doctors to accept that their own doctor–patient relationships are less than perfect. The idea that 'I am a good doctor, of course my patients take their tablets' has been taken almost as an article of faith. Any attempt to question this tenet implies a threat to this doctor's self-image and so has been resisted. Thus for many doctors what happens between prescription and consumption has been a blind-spot for enquiry: perfection has been easy and comforting to assume. A second reason for past neglect has been that this area is very difficult to research. In most aspects one is trying to measure a subjective, very human phenomenon. Scientists strive to produce 'hard' data, precisely and directly measuring reproducible phenomena under controlled conditions. Compliance data fail to meet the criteria for hard data on virtually any count. The act of compliance cannot normally be observed. Its absolute measurement is virtually impossible so that indirect measurements giving limited insight must be accepted. These measurements often depend on patient co-operation. The criteria for acceptable compliance vary with every drug, and are normally not known. Thus compliance must be a very 'soft' field. It may lack scientific glamour, despite its clinical importance. Recent studies at least enable a start to be made in analysing what happens after a prescription is written.

After a drug is prescribed, a sequence of events must occur before the drug becomes active in the body. A mistake in any link in this chain can reduce or abolish the drug's effectiveness. This chain of events is less simple than may appear at first glance. A correctly written prescription must be correctly dispensed with adequate instructions in an openable container. The patient must be mentally and physically able to read and comprehend the instructions and to take the tablets. He or she must wish to take the tablets. Last but not least, he or she must actually take the tablets. To improve the efficiency of drug prescribing, each of these steps needs analysis to see how efficient it is at present, how errors are made and how to reduce them.

Of the steps above, we know by far the most about compliance—the degree to which the patient decides to take the medication as prescribed. But before considering compliance, the sequence of steps between prescription and ingestion needs exploring in more detail, concentrating on areas most relevant to the elderly.

THE PRESCRIPTION ITSELF

The first step in the fulfilment of a prescription is the presentation of an accurate legible prescription to the dispensing pharmacist. Two types of error can occur here. The first is the most fundamental act of non-compliance—the patient fails to present the doctor's prescription for dispensing. Few studies appear to have been made of this problem, and even large reviews of compliance (Haynes *et al.*, 1979) ignore it completely. One study of 2000 prescriptions showed that 3% of prescriptions were not collected within 10 days (Hammel and William, 1964). Another rigorous study of non-compliance in outpatients noted that 24 of 356 prescriptions (i.e. 7%) were not presented for dispensing (Boyd *et al.*, 1974). A general practice study has also produced a figure of 7% (Waters *et al.*, 1976). In most compliance studies non-presentation is not commented on separately. One study has shown that the rate is lowest in diseases considered serious by the patient, but rose to 27% in prescriptions for minor analgesics (Waters *et al.*, 1976). The rate might also be higher where doctor–patient rapport is poor. However, this one study only highlights our lack of factual information.

The second group of potential errors lies in the prescription itself. It must be legible and contain no errors. Surprisingly, virtually no studies of this aspect of quality control in prescribing appear to have been published. One might wonder why this lacuna exists: perhaps doctors feel that such studies would pry too deeply into the privacy of prescribing, especially as studies would necessarily involve large numbers of doctors. One study in the pharmacy of a busy district general hospital (Nottingham City Hospital) (J. Gilby, unpublished observations) showed that some 3% of prescriptions were illegible. Pharmacists were unwilling to dispense a further 10% of prescriptions exactly as written. Of the 10%, about 6% were obvious errors (e.g. writing G instead of mg), which the pharmacist felt able to alter and dispense. In the other 4% the pharmacist felt they should discuss the prescription with the prescribing doctor. In half these cases (2%) serious toxicity could have occurred had they not done so.

A New Zealand study (Kellaway and McCrae, 1975) showed that 13% of patients received an inaccurately written prescription on leaving hospital. Even hospital inpatients may suffer from this problem: a study of drug use in five Boston hospitals showed that inpatient prescriptions were frequently incomplete (Borda *et al.*, 1967). In particular, instructions for route of administration were missing in 35–60% of prescriptions. This may have led to the substantial disparity seen between the doctor's prescription and doses recorded as dispensed in the nurses' files. This 1967 study was probably before the introduction of the more specific, accurate drug recording system used in hospitals today, so errors should be less common.

Discussions with hospital and dispensing pharmacists in several areas of Britain have produced estimates substantially similar to the Nottingham study, although most commercial dispensing pharmacists would discuss fewer than 4% of prescriptions with doctors. Thus the study is likely to be fairly typical: its figures suggesting that inaccurate prescribing is making a modest but real contribution to the misapplication of drugs.

Pharmacists reasonably alter obvious dosage mistakes on prescriptions without consulting the doctor. Sometimes, however, these alterations can be controversial and even dangerous. Macdonald (1977) noted two instances where pharmacists altered correct antituberculous drug prescriptions to give dangerously low doses, resulting in drug resistance.

The writing of a prescription by a person not medically qualified, with the doctor only signing it, could contribute to error. One large study in Swansea (Austin and Parish, 1976) showed that 10% of 65,000 GP prescriptions had been written by someone other than the prescribing doctor—presumably ancillary staff. For the elderly, the proportion thus written rose to 19%. Only half of these ancillary-written prescriptions contained adequate prescribing details, compared to three-quarters of prescriptions written by doctors. Use of this method of prescribing can only lower standards.

EFFECTIVE DISPENSING

After the presentation of the prescription, the next step is the dispensing of the drug in a well-labelled container that the patient is able to open. A well-labelled container must pass several tests: the label(s) must be legible, describe the dosage regimen in a way proven difficult to misunderstand, and have adequate identification details (drug name, method of administration, patient name, dispensary name, dispensing date, and, ideally, expiry date). How many of today's drug bottles pass muster? As in other areas, remarkably few good surveys have been done to answer this simple question. By far the best study is by Boyd *et al.* (1974) in Oklahoma. They found that only 31% of the 356 bottle labels examined included all the details above (plus purpose of drug). For instance, only 60% of labels showed the drug name despite the drug name being present on 98.9% of prescriptions. This discrepancy could well be a local problem. It seems odd that there does not appear to be a British study of labelling quality. It is difficult to imagine £1000 million being spent each year on a potentially dangerous consumer product without a body such as the British Standards Institute surveying the adequacy of instructions on how to use the machine, how to wire the plug, etc., but this is the position with drugs.

As well as providing all the identification details, a good label must state clearly the drug regimen in a manner difficult to misunderstand. Several studies have explored what patients understand by particular label instructions. The best study so far is by Herman (1973). She asked hospital outpatients at which hours of the day they planned to take their medication and compared these answers with their prescriptions. The study involved 381 prescription regimens. The 'take once daily' regimen was well understood. For the frequently used 'take twice (three times, four times) a day' the results were less reassuring. The mean intervals between the doses for the twice-daily regimens were 10.4 and 13.6 h, with 28% of patients having a dosage interval of more than 17 h.

For thrice-daily regimens the mean intervals were 4.5, 6.3, and 13.3 h (ideally at 8-h intervals). Some 23% of patients had a dosage interval of

3 h or less while 66% had one dosage interval of 12 h or longer. Similar results were seen with the four-times daily regimen. A similar study of thrice-daily spacing was undertaken by Alfredsson and Norell (1981). This only studied pilocarpine eyedrops but had the advantage of considering mainly geriatric patients (age range 56–90 years) and of studying the time of actual usage rather than the stated intention. The dosage spacing was still very uneven, with 10% of patients having a dosage interval of less than 3½ h and 40% having an interval of more than 11½ h.

Raynor (1978) studied the intended dosage spacing in 41 inpatients in Nottingham. He defined regular usage as every dose time being within 1 h of the ideal, i.e. 5–7 h for four times daily. Twice-daily regimens were regular in 90% of cases, four times daily in 68%, but thrice-daily doses were only correct in 3%. Ward prescribing practices may well have influenced these results. Comparable figures were, however, obtained by Mazzullo *et al.* (1974).

Hermann (1973) obtained 100% understanding when specific intervals were stated (take every 6 h). However, this claim was based on only 13 patients. Both Raynor (1978) and Mazzullo *et al.* (1974) studied this type of label in larger groups (41 and 67 patients respectively). This high degree of accuracy was not substantiated. By far the commonest mistake was to take every 6 hours for three doses only. Mazzullo *et al.* suggested that the patients perceived the 'day' as the hours of waking and spaced their drugs accordingly.

These studies all suggest that the commonly used wording for dosage instructions is widely misunderstood, resulting in great variations in the times of administration. Specified intervals are probably better than the thrice-daily format. In reality, does this matter? Dosage frequencies are allocated during the development of the drug, usually on the basis of the serum half-life rather than on the therapeutic half-life. Many drugs are active for longer than conventional prescribing practice would suggest. Methyldopa is usually prescribed thrice daily, whereas a twice-daily dose is just as effective (Hollifield and Slaton, 1978; Wilson *et al.*, 1979). One recent study has indicated that good control of hypertension can be achieved with a single night-time dose (Wright *et al.*, 1976). The implications of such findings on prescribing patterns in the elderly are enormous. Frequency modification trials are rare, so the minimum frequency for efficacy is simply not known for most drugs. For a few drugs, dosage spacing may well be very important, e.g. pilocarpine eyedrops for glaucoma, anti-arrhythmic drugs, and some anti-epileptics. In the main, doses irregularly spaced through the day are probably not very important. It is, however, important to find if the overall frequency of administation can be reduced.

Nevertheless, to continue to prescribe drugs with labels which we know are widely misunderstood is clearly unsatisfactory. Trials are needed of other types of wording such as suggesting specific times—'take at about 8 a.m., 2 p.m., and 10 p.m.'.

Other aspects of labelling can give rise to misunderstanding. Potentially the most important is the direction 'take before meals'. 42% of patients thought this meant immediately before meals, 42% about ½ h before meals, 12% about 1 h before food and 5% any time between meals (Raynor, 1978). This variation can influence the drug absorption and is discussed further in Chapter 2. Mazzullo *et al.* (1974) found that 91% of patients took their medication correctly with the direction 'take 30 minutes before meals on an empty stomach'. This direction is clearly better. Some drugs, such as nitrofurantoin, need to be taken during meals to reduce nausea and increase absorption. Similar misunderstandings due to vague wording occurred with this timing, with only 33% of patients taking their therapy at the correct time (Mazzullo *et al.*, 1974).

One would expect the label 'take as directed' to be frequently misunderstood, as it is vague and relies exclusively on the patient's memory of the interview with his doctor. This recall has been shown both to be poor and prone to confusion. Powell *et al.* (1973) compared the patient's immediate recall of this 'as directed' regimen with what the prescribing doctor said he said. In 38% of cases there was a significant difference. This large figure would doubtless grow even higher with time, as the memory of the interview fades into the distance and becomes overlaid with more recent events.

We thus know that many of the instructions we write on our drug labels are misinterpreted. This link in the prescribing chain is relatively weak. Pharmaceutical bodies place considerable stress on precision in prescription writing, and issue doctors with the British National Formulary, *Prescribers' Journal*, etc. to give exact doses, timing, and so on. A massive effort rightly goes into making the doctor–pharmacist link in the chain as strong as possible. But a chain is only as strong as its weakest link. If the pharmacist–patient link is already much weaker than the doctor–pharmacist link, then it would seem both sensible and efficient for prescribing authorities to put more effort into trying to improve the quality of the labelling. What is the use of all that prescribing precision if up to half the patients do not understand the instructions? One way forward would be to have trials of improved wording. That wording could then be made the norm by putting an 'opt-out' box on NHS prescriptions, like the present 'NP' box for ensuring bottle labelling with the drug name. All prescriptions would be dispensed with the most efficient labelling available for the designated regimen unless the prescriber wrote otherwise. If we are at all serious about getting patients to take drugs properly, then this would seem a sensible step.

The efficacy of various types of wording is summarized in Table 12.1.

Table 12.1   Patients' comprehension of wording on drug labels

---

Well understood
Take once daily
Take at about 8 a.m. and 8 p.m.
    8 a.m., 2 p.m., and 10 p.m.
    8 a.m., 1 p.m., 6 p.m., and 10 p.m., etc.
Take 30 minutes before meals on an empty stomach
Take during meals
Take every __ hours as needed for (symptom)

Moderately poorly understood
Take every 6 hours
    8 hours
Take twice daily

Poorly understood
Take three times daily
   four times daily
Take with meals
Take for fluid retention
Take as directed

Labels must also be legible. Very little information is available on legibility. This is a particular problem in the elderly, where diminished visual acuity is common. Raynor (1978) noted that prescription instructions from local chemists were typewritten in only 27% of cases. However, 63% of patients in the study would have preferred typewritten labels. Beanland (1975) has suggested an attractive system of labelling, with a typewritten label giving identification (name, drug, tablet strength, date, etc.) on one side of the bottle and a printed label with instructions on the other side. If this became widespread, labelling quality would rise considerably.

All the labelling problems above are likely to cause difficulty for the elderly. Their poor eyesight will increase the legibility problems, especially with handwritten labels. They are more likely than younger groups to be on several drugs, making correct identification vital and the integration of schedules more difficult when the instructions are poorly understood. They are more likely to be on long-term therapy, with the high risk of repeat prescriptions carrying the vague 'as before' or 'as directed' labels. It is essential that the instructions are also tailored to the mental capacity of the recipient. Considerable success can be obtained by colour coding on the bottles (Macdonald *et al.*, 1977).

PHYSICAL OPENING PROBLEMS

The old are more likely to have problems opening their drug containers. This takes co-ordination, muscle power, and joint flexibility as well as a modicum of eyesight and mental orientation. All these facets tend to decline in the elderly. Probably the most frequent difficulty arises from arthritis and tremor causing co-ordination problems. Few surveys of this have been made. Lane *et al.* (1971) note that 5% of their sample (mean age 61) had some difficulty in opening their screw-top containers.

Two new developments are increasing physical opening problems: the use of blister packs and childproof containers.

Davidson (1973) made a well-analysed study of the speed with which 49 geriatric inpatients could remove a tablet from various types of container. The three types of strip-foil pack produced the worst results of all. For the best of these packs (a push-through bubble pack), only 16% of patients could remove a tablet within 10 seconds, and 30% failed completely. The results were markedly worse for patients with poor vision, poor manual dexterity or poor mental function. Fogden *et al.* (1976) questioned 92 outpatients at a rheumatology clinic who had used a blister pack —36% did not like them. The main reasons were that they were difficult to open, the tablets broke on opening, or they came out so quickly that they fell on the floor. Outpatients with rheumatoid arthritis found opening particularly difficult. A more detailed study of 30 inpatients with rheumatoid arthritis showed that none of them liked blister packs. Those with mild hand changes could open the packs with difficulty, but 30% of those with more severe hand changes could not open the packs at all. Most of the patients who could open the packs had to press the tablet out on to the table then pick the tablet up. These studie suggest that blister packaging will make access to tablets much more difficult for many old people—an entirely unnecessary extra burden. Despite these studies, the Medicines Commission (1974) concluded that blister packs could be opened by most elderly people. Their evidence for this view was not stated. No studies have been made of the effect of these packs on compliance, but it cannot be beneficial.

Child-resistant containers are deliberately made difficult to open—allegedly just for children. They have been mandatory for children's aspirin and paracetamol bottles since 1976. Their introduction has been remarkably successful in reducing the incidence of accidental analgesic overdoses in children both in Britain (Sibert *et al.*, 1977) and America (Scherz, 1970). In the British studies, aspirin overdoses were reduced to one-quarter of their previous level. After this success, demands for the extension of child-resistant containers to other drugs have been growing (Craft and Sibert, 1979). The Pharmaceutical Society have recently suggested that all tablets be routinely dispensed in these containers.

There is, however, a price to be paid for all this 'child-proofing'. Several studies have shown that many old people find these containers very difficult to open. Lane *et al.* (1971) made a thorough controlled study of how these containers were actually used by patients. Their study included people up to the age of 87 years. They found that 16% of child-proof containers were improperly closed, compared to 2% of ordinary bottles. 10% of child-proof containers had to be opened by a person other than the patient. Only 30% of patients had no difficulty with child-proof containers, compared with 70% experiencing moderate to severe difficulty. Patient compliance, measured by pill counting, was markedly worse with child-proof containers. A similar study in Virginia (Myers, 1977) produced similar results, together with a horrifying list of tools used by 46% of patients to open the containers—including a wrench!

In America a well-structure telephone survey of 636 households has shown that 89% of families had child-resistant containers at home (McIntire *et al.*, 1977). Misuse of containers was frequent, rising with age. Some 33% of respondents over 60 years said they could not use them properly. They either changed the container or left the top off. Only 3% admitted to stopping using the drug because of difficulty in opening the container. A direct survey by Sherman (1978) showed that 60% of elderly people living at home had trouble opening child-resistant containers. In Britain, Bellamy *et al.* (1981) assessed the three commonest types of child-resistant containers on 74 geriatric day-hospital patients. Only 54% could open the easiest container. However, only 3% of patients could generate sufficient torque to close even the easiest container.

One large chain of British dispensing chemists (Boots) has made a study of 255 patients of all ages with experience of child-resistant con-

214

Table 12.2   Summary of how to reduce packaging problems in the
elderly

Prescriber
Is your prescription really necessary?
Be sure your prescription is clearly legible
Write it yourself
Re-read it to eliminate errors
Write clear directions for timing (see Table 12.1)
Avoid blister packs
Avoid child-resistant containers unless patient lives with a child

Pharmacist
Use typed labels
Use a clear label format (consider the Beanland system)
Check that the patient can open the container
Avoid blister packs
Avoid child-resistant containers
Avoid coloured bottles

---

tainers (Silverman, 1976). Some 21% could not open them and 13%
could not close these containers.

It is also worth while to note in passing that misuse of child-resistant
containers by younger subjects in these studies is not uncommon. The
largest study (McIntire *et al.*, 1977) showed that 23% of subjects aged
30–60 years were unable to open the containers properly. In this younger
age group, a high proportion of those unable to open the container
stopped the drug completely.

So the catch-phrase 'child-proof means granny-proof' has a ring of
truth to it. We have a dilemma: child overdoses or reduced elderly compliance? Both can cause death. The overall advantages of dispensing in
these containers to old people is debatable. The safety of children is
important, but inadequate therapy can be lethal. Relatively few old
people live with their grandchildren (8% in the USA). Perhaps the best
compromise would be to make these containers truly optional for the
elderly by asking if they are required at the point of dispensing or mark-
ing the prescription accordingly when the prescriber has the patient with
him and can look at his dexterity.

These two 'improvements' have made taking medication harder for
the old. Another idea has been the use of packs designed to remind
patients to take their drugs. Several models are available (Dosett,
Doseaid, and Pill Wheel). The central problem again is access to the
drugs. The compartments are small. Access needs space for two fingers
and pill in each compartment or the ability to invert the pack without all

the other tablets falling out. In practice, access is difficult even for the dexterous, and most elderly patients usually find them fiddly and inconvenient.

REFERENCES AND BIBLIOGRAPHY

Alfredsson, L. S. and Norell, S. E. (1981) Spacing between doses on a thrice-daily regimen. *Brit. Med. J.*, **282**, 1036.

Austin, R. and Parish, P. (1976) Prescriptions written by ancillary staff. *J. Roy. Coll. Gen. Pract.* (suppl.), **26**, 44–9.

Beanland, W. A. (1975) A new approach to labelling. *Pharmaceut. J.*, **214**, 507.

Bellamy, K. A. *et al.* (1981) A study of child resistance and geriatric acceptability to a range of dispensing containers. *Brit. J. Pharm. Prac.*, **2**, 4–11.

Borda, I. *et al.* (1967) Studies of drug usage in five Boston hospitals. *JAMA*, **202**, 506–10.

Boyd, J. R. *et al.* (1974) Drug defaulting: an analysis of non-compliance patterns. *Am. J. Hosp. Pharm.*, **31**, 485–91.

Craft, W. A. and Sibert, J. R. (1979) Preventive effects of C.R.C.S. *Pharm. J.*, **222**, 593.

Davidson, J. R. (1973) Presentation and packaging of drugs for the elderly. *J. Hosp. Pharm.*, **31**, 180–4.

Fogden, J. *et al.* (1976) The packaging of antirheumatic drugs. *Occup. Ther.*, **39**, 32.

Gilby, J. G. (1978) Unpublished observations.

Hammel, R. W. and William, P. O. (1964) Do patients receive prescribed medication? *J. Am. Pharm. Assoc.*, **NS4**, 331–3 and 337.

Haynes, R. B., Taylor, D. W., and Sackett, D. L. (eds) (1979), *Compliance in Health Care*. Johns Hopkins University Press, Baltimore.

Hermann, F. (1973) The outpatient prescription label as a source of medication errors. *Am. J. Hosp. Pharm.*, **30**, 155–9.

Hollifield, J. W. and Slaton, P. E. (1978) Effectiveness of twice-daily methyldopa in essential hypertension. *J. Tenn. Med. Assoc.*, **71**, 337.

Kellaway, G. S. M. and McCrae, E. (1975) Non-compliance and errors of drug administration in patients discharged from acute medical wards. *N.Z. Med. J.*, **81**, 506–10.

Lane, M. F. *et al.* (1971) Child-resistant medical containers: experience in the home. *Am. J. Pub. Health*, **61**, 1861–8.

Macdonald, E. T. *et al.* (1977) Improving drug compliance after hospital discharge. *Brit. Med. J.*, **2**, 618–21.

Macdonald, J. B. (1977) Mycobacterium tuberculosis resistance: a clinical survey. *Thorax*, **32**, 1.

McIntire, M. S. *et al.* (1977) Safety packaging—what does the public think? *Am. J. Pub. Health*, **69**, 169–71.

Mazzullo, J. M. *et al.* (1974) Variations in interpretation of prescription instructions. *JAMA*, **227**, 929–31.

Medicines Commission (1974). *The presentation of medicines in relation to child safety*. HMSO, London.

Myers, C. E. (1977) Patient experiences with child-resistant containers. *Am. J. Hosp. Pharm.*, **34**, 255–8.

Powell, J. R. *et al.* (1973) Inadequately written prescriptions. *JAMA*, **226**, 999.

Raynor, D. K. (1978) *Study of Patient Non-comprehension*. Trent Regional Health Authority Preregistration Pharmacy Graduate Project.

Scherz, R. G. (1970) Prevention of childhood poisoning: a community problem. *Paediat. Clin. N.A.*, **17**, 713–27.

Sherman, F. (1978) Geriatric generic prescribing form. *N.Y. State Med. J.*, **78**, 1293.

Sibert, J. R. *et al.* (1977) Child-resistant packaging and accidental childhood poisoning. *Lancet*, **2**, 289.

Silverman, B. (1976) Experience with child-resistant containers. *Pharm. J.*, **216**, 297–8.

Waters, W. H. R. *et al.* (1976) Undispensed prescriptions in a mining general practice. *Brit. Med. J.*, **1**, 1062–3.

Wilson, L. *et al.* (1979) Twice-daily methyldopa. *Med. J. Aust.*, **1**, 363–4.

Wright, J. M. *et al.* (1976) Antihypertensive efficacy of single daily dose methyldopa. *Clin. Pharmacol. Ther.*, **20**, 733.

Chapter 13

The incidence of non-compliance

Studying compliance is only relevant if non-compliance is commonplace. If virtually all patients took their tablets religiously, the subject would rightly fade into obscurity. So we need to know the size of the problem. The literature is replete with over 500 studies measuring compliance. These studies cover a massive spectrum of drugs, diseases, ages, samples, and compliance definitions, so getting a reliable view is not easy. Many papers offer only short-term assessment of a sample of patients attending one clinic at a particular time. The technique is convenient but inadequate, so many compliance studies need to be interpreted warily.

Probably the best method of assembling a patient sample to assess patient compliance is to follow prospectively all the patients in an area just starting a specific treatment for one disease. Every single patient needs to be followed up—non-attenders included. A survey of clinic attenders is a survey of survivors, and is likely to over-estimate compliance. Ideally non-compliance should not be defined as failing to take some arbitrary percentage of medication, but full details of the distribution of compliance rates supplied. Very few compliance studies reach these standards, and in only about 10% of published studies is the sampling well defined and reasonably good.

Other factors can also distort reported compliance rates:

(1) Doctors investigating compliance are interested in the subject: their interest is likely to have led to greater self-awareness and above-average compliance rate among their patients.
(2) Most compliance studies are from large academically orientated hospitals in big cities. They may well attract slightly more dedicated patients. This is particularly likely to be true in North America.
(3) Bad news sells newspapers. Papers showing dramatically poor compliance rates may be seen as more interesting and may well stand more chance of publication than articles showing good compliance.
(4) Definitions of non-compliance vary widely. For example, studies based on interview or pill-counting have defined non-compliance as taking less than 100% (Closson and Kikugawa, 1975; Hemminki and Heikkila, 1975); 90% (Drury *et al.*, 1976); 85% (Parkin *et al.*, 1976); 80% (Marshall and Barritt, 1977); or 50% (Macdonald *et al.*, 1977).

Despite these problems it is possible to get an approximate estimate of overall compliance by looking at well-conducted studies. Very few studies have assessed only geriatric patients, although in many other trials they make up a substantial proportion of the patients. The relevant studies are detailed in Table 13.1.

Hemminki and Heikkila (1975) interviewed 217 elderly people living in old people's homes in Helsinki. Patients admitted poor compliance for 28% of prescribed drugs, and in a further 2% admitted using excessive doses. Overall, 53% of patients had at least one drug with poor compliance. The highest non-compliance rates were for psychotropic drugs (49%) and analgesics (79%). Gibson and O'Hare (1968) interviewed 273 geriatric patients at home in Glasgow; 15% admitted that their drugs were not taken fully. Compliance was distinctly better where adequate supervision of drug-taking was possible. Our own study in Nottingham (Macdonald *et al.*, 1977), using pill counting, showed that 48% of elderly patients were taking less than half their prescribed tablets 6 weeks after hospital discharge. Also 26% were taking at least twice the prescribed number of tablets.

Schwartz *et al.* (1962) noted non-compliance in 59% of elderly outpatients in New York, and 26% of the errors were deemed potentially serious. Unfortunately, the definition of error included the use of non-prescribed drugs and inaccurate knowledge of tablet purpose, so the figures are not exactly comparable with other studies. Almost identical results came from a smaller study in Seattle (Neely and Patrick, 1968).

Parkin *et al.* (1976) studied compliance after hospital discharge. Their patients were not specifically geriatric, but had a mean age of 66.2 years. Ten days after hospital discharge, 26% of patients had less than 85% compliance by pill counting. In our own study (Macdonald *et al.*, 1977) we defined compliance as taking between 50% and 200% of prescribed tablets. Even using these generous criteria, only 23% of uncounselled patients and 53% of counselled patients were complying 12 weeks after their discharge from hospital.

These five studies (summarized in Table 13.1) show a wide range, with the more rigorous studies perhaps tending to show poorer compliance rates. It is interesting to contrast these results in old people with those obtained in good studies in other age groups. These are summarized in Table 13.2.

Hedstrand and Aberg (1976) reviewed the notes of 2322 men noted to be hypertensive in a community survey, then started on therapy. One year later 94% were still visiting their doctor and on treatment, but by 2 years the figure had dropped to 65% and by 3 years to 34%—a frighten-

Table 13.1 Incidence of compliance among elderly subjects

Reference	Study group	Drugs	Measurement technique	Compliance definition	Compliance (%)
Hemminki and Heikkila (1975)	217 patients in homes for the elderly	Various (long-term)	Interview	Taking drugs correctly	70
Gibson and O'Hare (1968)	273 patients seen on domiciliary visits	Various (long-term)	Interview	Taking drugs correctly	85
Schwartz *et al.* (1962)	178 outpatients	Various	Interview	Taking drugs correctly and knowing drug purpose	41
Parkin *et al.* (1976)	130 patients recently discharged from hospital	Various	Interview and pill counting	Taking $\geq$85%	74
Macdonald *et al.* (1977)	60 patients recently discharged from hospital	Various	Pill counting	Taking $\geq$50% or <200% of drugs	25

Table 13.2   Incidence of compliance in well-documented studies involving adults

Reference	Study group	Drugs	Measurement technique	Compliance definition	Compliance (%)
Hedstrand and Aberg (1976)	2322 hypertensive men in the community	Hypotensives	Review of notes	Still visiting doctor and on treatment	94 at 1 year 65 at 2 years 34 at 3 years
Langfeld (1973)	185 previously diagnosed hypertensives	Hypotensives	Questionnaire	Still visiting doctor and on treatment	69
Sackett *et al.* (1975)	230 hypertensive steelworkers	Hypotensives	Pill count	Taking $\geqslant$80% of drugs	53
Hulka *et al.* (1976)	357 patients with diabetes or heart failure	Various	Interview	Taking drugs correctly	42
Hogarty *et al.* (1973)	374 schizophrenic outpatients	Tranquillizers	Interview	Taking drugs correctly	42
Lipman *et al.* (1965)	254 outpatients in tranquillizer trial	Tranquillizers	Pill count	Taking $\geqslant$75% of drugs	54

ingly low figure. Langfeld (1973) sent questionnaires to patients found to be hypertensive before surgery. Of those previously known to be hypertensive and to have been started on antihypertensive drugs, 69% were still taking their drugs. Sackett *et al.* (1975) measured compliance by pill count in hypertensive steelworkers. They found that only 53% were taking 80% or more of their medication 6 months after starting treatment.

In a very detailed interview study of 357 patients with diabetes or heart failure, Hulka *et al.* (1976) found that only 42% claimed to be taking their drugs correctly. This is one of the most refined studies ever made of compliance, with meticulous analysis of a wide range of underlying factors. Curiously, exactly the same percentage of compliance was obtained by Hogarty *et al.* (1973) using a similar definition and technique to assess schizophrenic outpatients. Pill counts were used to assess outpatient tranquillizer usage by Lipman *et al.* (1965); 54% of patients were taking more than 75% of their medication.

These studies (Table 13.2) produce a wide range of compliance. This is only to be expected since definitions, clinical settings, and measurement techniques vary considerably. The unweighted mean of the compliance rates in Table 13.2 is 49%. So it seems reasonable to assume that on long-term treatment compliance rates will be about 50%. (Many other less rigorous studies produce similar figures.) Compliance on short-term medication is only slightly better.

Among elderly patients, the average compliance for Table 13.1 is 59%. This includes some less rigorous studies, so need to be treated with a little caution. Does it signify that older people comply better? One large review (Haynes *et al.*, 1979) examined the effect of age on compliance in various studies. Some 18 studies have found that compliance improves with age, with eight studies showing a decline with age and 64 studies showing no effect of age on compliance. This broad-based study suggests that age probably influences compliance very little. If there is any trend at all, it is towards a marginal improvement in compliance with increasing age.

Thus non-compliance is massive on long-term therapy. Half the patients started on long-term therapy do not take their tablets regularly. The implications of this simple statement are so huge that we almost need to take a step back from this conclusion to take it in fully. Here are a few immediate repercussions:

(1) Tens of millions of pounds are spent every year on drugs that are not used. What happens to these millions of tablets? How many are consumed after their expiry date? How many are used by friends or relatives?

(2) Either too many tablets are prescribed and the public wisely rejects many of them, or there is a large reservoir of ill health in the community caused by non-compliance. We need to know which is the case. Either way the doctor needs to prune down his prescription numbers to the really essential, then make better efforts to see that those essential drugs actually get taken.

(3) If normal compliance is so poor, then compliance analysis should be part of every drug trial. There is reason to suppose that compliance in trials tends to be higher because of the increased attention given to the patient. Nevertheless, good compliance can no longer be assumed. Poor compliance tends to reduce the effect of a regimen: in how many trials has poor compliance concealed genuine differences between regimens?

The discovery of such widespread non-compliance makes the analysis of factors associated with poor compliance important in order to identify 'high-risk' groups. Literally dozens of such factors have been investigated, of which the most important are:

The patient

Age

As noted above, very little association with a minimal tendency to improve with age.

Sex

Most studies have found no association.

Social class

Compliance seems to improve slightly with rising social class, although many reports have found no association.

Education

Although quite a few studies have shown that compliance is better in highly educated patients, the majority of studies have found no correlation.

Social isolation

This factor (potentially very important in the elderly) has been little studied, but several papers have shown better compliance when drug-taking is supervised. Thus social isolation may well be associated with poor compliance in the elderly.

Race, cultural and religious backgrounds

No association.

The illness

Diagnosis

Past studies split evenly. About half find that compliance is better in some types of disease than others, while half find no association. Psychiatric patients appear to have poorer compliance than other patients and of the psychiatric diagnoses, schizophrenia, personality disorders, and paranoid features are associated with particularly poor compliance.

Severity

Here a striking conclusion has been found by virtually all studies. There is NO association between severity of disease and compliance. This conclusion is the opposite of what might be expected by 'common sense'. It also demonstrates that compliance research is not merely the flat-footed measurement of the obvious. So 'common sense' is no substitute for scientific enquiry in this field, as in any other.

Duration of the disease

Neither disease duration nor previous hospital admission for it affects compliance.

Symptoms

No study has ever found that increasing severity of symptoms improves compliance. Indeed, four papers have shown decreasing compliance with worsening symptoms. The four studies are of high quality, cover a wide range of conditions, and constitute formidable evidence. A further three papers have shown no association. This again runs counter to 'common sense' but fits in well with the influence of disease severity (see above).

Disability

Despite a few studies showing no association, the balance of the evidence is that increasing disability improves compliance. At first sight this seems inconsistent with the effect of symptoms (see above). It is probably simply a reflection of the increased medical attention and supervision given to the more disabled patients. This strongly improves compliance.

Clinical improvement

No effect on compliance.

Other concurrent illness

No effect.

The regimen

Route of administration

Parenteral administration under direct supervision has been exceptionally successful in ensuring high compliance rates. Using this method outside hospital is normally only feasible if the drug can be made in a long-acting form. Supervised parenteral administration has been successfully used in the prophylaxis of rheumatic fever and treating tuberculosis (especially drug-resistant non-compliant patients). Its most spectacular success is, of course, in using long-acting depot preparations of phenothiazine in the treatment of schizophrenia. The very poor compliance rate for self-injected insulin in diabetics (Watkins *et al.*, 1967) shows that it is the direct supervision, not the parenteral route, that is the important factor.

There are no studies comparing other routes, e.g. rectal versus oral, for similar drugs.

Type of drug

Compliance seems to vary little between different types of oral drug given for the same disease. But this is not true between drugs given for different diseases. Several studies have shown that cardiac and diabetic drugs have the highest compliance rates (80–90% in those studies). Hypotensives and diuretics come next (60–70%), with relatively low compliance rates for more symptomatic drugs such as sedatives, hypnotics, analgesics, and antacids (40–50%).

If diagnosis has little effect on compliance, and different drugs for the same condition have similar compliance, then why does compliance vary between different classes of drugs? No-one knows, but it may be that patients perceive some types of disease as being more 'serious'. If they are seen as greater threats to health, compliance may be higher. Also these diseases may be more closely supervised.

Duration of treatment

Virtually all studies agree that the longer a given regimen is prescribed, the lower the compliance. This contrasts with the lack of effect on compliance shown by disease duration rather than treatment duration.

Number of drugs prescribed

The number of types of treatment a patient has to take has an important effect on compliance—the more types, the worse the compliance. This appears to be particularly true in the elderly, where virtually all researchers have found that three or four drug types is the effective upper limit. Above this number compliance declines catastrophically.

Frequency of dosing

Drug advertisements often claim that reducing dose frequency will automatically improve compliance. However, the truth of this 'common-sense' statement is far from proven. Three good studies (Parkin *et al.*, 1976; McInnis, 1970; Lima *et al.*, 1976) have shown no correlation between compliance and the number of drug doses per day. Two other studies (Brand *et al.*, 1977; Gatley, 1968) have shown a substantial drop in compliance as dosage frequency increased from once to four times daily. This point needs further clarification.

Dose

The effect of dose *per se* has been little studied and no firm conclusions are available.

Side-effects

Contrary to popular belief, side-effects seem to have relatively little effect on compliance. Studies have found no difference in frequency of side-effects between compliers and non-compliers. Side-effects are only rarely mentioned by non-compliers as reasons for their non-compliance.

The effects of these features of the patient, the disease, and the regimen on compliance are summarized in Table 13.3. Other aspects, such as short clinic waiting times and individual clinic appointments, improve compliance with appointments. So they will probably reduce dropout rates and indirectly improve overall drug compliance.

In summary, many of the factors affecting compliance have predictable effects. It is, however, important to remember those which are not as expected. The severity of his illness has NO effect on the patient's compliance, nor has the length of his illness. As his symptoms grow more severe he is likely to become less compliant, not more compliant. Side-effects will not affect his compliance.

Table 13.3　Factors affecting drug compliance

	Effect on compliance		
	Positive	Negative	No effect
The patient	Age (slight) Education	Low social class Social isolation	Sex Race
The illness	Disability	Severity of symptoms Psychiatric illness	Severity of illness Disease duration Clinical improvement Concurrent illness
The regimen	Supervised parenteral administration Cardiac drugs Diabetic drugs	Duration of therapy Number of drugs Frequency of doses Symptomatic drugs	Side-effects

REFERENCES

Brand, F. *et al.* (1977) Effect of economic barriers to medical care on patient compliance. *Pub. Health Rep.*, **92**, 72–8.

Closson, R. and Kikugawa, C. (1975) Non-compliance varies with drug class. *Hospitals*, **49**, 89–93.

Drury, V. *et al.* (1976) Following advice in general practice. *Prev. Med.*, **5**, 414–24.

Gatley, M. S. (1968) To be taken as directed. *J. R. Coll. Gen. Pract.*, **16**, 39–44.

Gibson, I. and O'Hare, M. (1968) Prescription of drugs for old people at home. *Gerontol. Clin.*, **10**, 271–80.

Haynes, R. B., Taylor, D. W., and Sackett, D. L. (eds) (1979) *Compliance in Health Care*, p. 460. Johns Hopkins University Press, Baltimore.

Hedstrand, H. and Aberg, H. (1976) Treatment of hypertension in middle-aged men. *Acta Med. Scand.*, **199**, 281–8.

Hemminki, E. and Heikkila, J. (1975) Elderly people's compliance with prescriptions and quality of medication. *Scand. J. Soc. Med.*, **3**, 87–92.

Hogarty, G. E. *et al.* (1973) Drug and sociotherapy in the aftercare of schizophrenic patients: one year relapse rates. *Arch. Gen. Psychiat.*, **28**, 54–64.

Hulka, B. *et al.* (1976) Communications, compliance and concordance between physicians and patients with prescribed medication. *Am. J. Publ. Health*, **66**, 647–53.

Langfeld, B. S. (1973) Hypertension: deficient care of the medically served. *Ann. Intern. Med.*, **78**, 19–23.

Lima, J. *et al.* (1976) Compliance with short-term antimicrobial therapy. *Paediatrics*, **57**, 383–6.

Lipman, R. S. *et al.* (1965) Neurotics who fail to take their drugs. *Brit. J. Psychiat.*, **3**, 1043–9.

Macdonald, E. T. *et al.* (1977) Improving drug compliance after hospital discharge. *Br. Med. J.*, **2**, 618–21.

McInnis, J. K. (1970) Do patients take antituberculosis drugs? *Am. J. Nurs.*, **70**, 2152–3.

Marshall, A. and Barritt, D. W. (1977) Drug compliance in hypertensive patients. *Brit. Med. J.*, **1**, 1278–9.

Neely, E. and Patrick, M. L. (1968) Problems of aged persons taking medication at home. *Nurs. Res.*, **17**, 52–5.

Parkin, D. M. *et al.* (1976) Deviation from prescribed drug treatment after discharge from hospital. *Brit. Med. J.*, **2**, 686–8.

Sackett, D. L. *et al.* (1975) Randomised clinical trials of strategies for improving medication compliance in hypertension. *Lancet*, **1**, 1205–7.

Schwartz, D. *et al.* (1962) Medication errors made by elderly chronically ill patients. *Am. J. Publ. Health*, **52**, 2018–29.

Watkins, J. D. *et al.* (1967) A study of diabetic patients at home. *Am. J. Publ. Health*, **57**, 452–9.

Chapter 14

Methods of improving compliance

Since non-compliance is widespread, finding ways of improving compliance becomes important. We must look again at the chain of events from prescription to ingestion.

PRESCRIBING AND DISPENSING

Useful measures are summarized in Table 14.1 and most of the data underlying the following suggestions have been presented in Chapter 12. For the prescribing doctor the first question must be—Is your prescription really necessary? Compliance could even be counter-productive on an unneeded prescription. Then the prescription must be accurate and legible. Doctors are famed for illegible writing, and an estimated 3% of prescriptions are totally illegible. The proportion of prescriptions where virtual illegibility leads to dispensing problems may well be even higher. So clear writing really matters. Are we all sure that other people can always read every word we write? They have to, on a prescription. Mistakes seem to occur in about 10% of prescriptions. Over half of these are so obvious (e.g. g instead of mg) that pharmacists feel able to correct them without consultation. For other dubious cases it would help to make consultation between the pharmacist and the general practitioner as easy as possible. One way would be to always include the practice telephone number in the doctor's stamp on the prescription.

Ancillary staff are frequently used to write prescriptions. This practice is well shown to reduce prescribing quality. Obviously it is to be avoided: there might even be a case for the NHS to refuse to accept these prescriptions for payment.

Badly worded prescription details are misunderstood by a frighteningly high proportion of patients. Table 14.2 gives details of which exact wording on drug labels is best understood.

The pharmacist has a sizeable role to play in reducing dispensing problems. Most patients prefer labels to be typed rather than hand-written. This is particularly true for old people who have poor vision. Beanland (1975) has proposed a system of mainly printed labels which would be a great asset if widely used. Many old people prefer clear to amber bottles, to aid tablet identification. Why not offer this option? Child-resistant

Table 14.1   Methods of reducing prescribing and dispensing problems in the elderly

---

Prescriber
Is your prescription really necessary?
Write it yourself
Make sure it is legible
Put in all the details needed (see BNF 1981 (1), p. 4)
Re-read it to eliminate errors
Write clear directions for timing, etc. (see Table 14.2)
Avoid drugs only available in blister packs

Pharmacist
Use typed labels
Use a clear label format (consider the Beanland system)
Avoid blister packs
Avoid child-resistant containers unless the patient wants one
Avoid coloured bottles
Check that the patient can open and close the container

Table 14.2   To improve clarity in drug labelling

Use
Take once daily
Take at about 8 a.m. and 8 p.m.
        8 a.m., 2 p.m., and 10 p.m.
        8 a.m., 1 p.m., 6 p.m., and 10 p.m.
Take 30 minutes before meals on an empty stomach
Take during meals
Take every __ hours as needed for (symptom)

Try to avoid
Take every 6 hours
        8 hours
Take twice daily

Avoid
Take three times daily
    four times daily
Take with meals
Take for fluid retention
Take as directed
Take as before

---

containers and blister packs have been clearly shown to be much harder for people to open, and compliance is definitely lower for drugs in such containers. Perhaps the best system would be for the pharmacist to offer each old person the option of a child-resistant container but to otherwise dispense in an ordinary screw-top bottle, and to avoid blister packs for the elderly patient if at all possible. It always helps to check that an old person can actually open and close the dispensed container.

NON-COMPREHENSION

After receiving his clearly labelled, easy-to-open bottle the patient may still misunderstand his regimen. Parkin *et al.* (1976) showed that non-comprehension caused deviations more than twice as commonly as wilful non-compliance in a group of oldish patients leaving hospital. Non-comprehension is important, so how can it be improved? Parkin *et al.* showed that dose frequency had virtually no effect on non-comprehension, but number of drugs had a powerful effect where more than three drug types were prescribed. So cutting down on the number of drugs should help that patient to master his regimen. In our own study in Nottingham (Macdonald *et al.*, 1977) we looked at the effect of counselling on the incidence of regimen non-comprehension. Before discharge each geriatric patient was visited by the ward pharmacist, who explained the regimen and made sure the patient understood it fully. Twelve weeks after their discharge 68% of the counselled patients could recall their regimens correctly, while only 42% of the uncounselled patients could do so. So detailed instruction improves regimen understanding for 12 weeks at least. Sadly, this appears to be the only controlled study of any technique to specifically improve non-comprehension. Most studies of methods for improving compliance do not differentiate non-comprehension from wilful non-compliance. For practical purposes we have to consider the two together and will call their sum 'adherence'.

ADHERENCE

Many methods of improving adherence to drug regimens have been tried, and the basic conclusions can now be stated with some confidence. Techniques assessed have included:

Educating patients about their disease

At least six good studies have examined the effect of teaching patients about their disease and how it is best managed. Methods have included individual instruction (Hecht, 1974); demonstrations and lectures (Bowen *et al.*, 1961; Tagliacozzo *et al.*, 1974); and programmed instruction (Sackett *et al.*, 1975; Etzwiler and Robb, 1972). The diseases studied were mainly diabetes and hypertension. The methods were all vigorously applied and were very effective in improving patients' knowledge of their disease. But none made any difference at all to regimen adherence or clinical outcome. So the conclusion for improving adherence is clear: patient disease education is useless.

Educating patients about their regimen

In contrast to disease education, regimen education appears fairly successful. It seems particularly useful for short-term regimens such as courses of antibiotics. Several of the most rigorous studies have been on paediatric prescribing, but at least two cogent studies in adults (Sharpe and Mikeal, 1974; Linkewich *et al.*, 1974) have shown substantially improved adherence to short antibiotic courses after verbal and written instructions.

Teaching patients about their regimens is less effective for long-term medications. Several studies (Clinite and Kabat, 1976; Malahy, 1966; Rehder *et al.*, 1980) have shown little or no improvement for pharmacists or nurses teaching patients on chronic regimens about their medication. However, Cole and Emmanuel (1971) showed a distinct improvement in adherence 2 weeks after counselling. Our own study (Macdonald *et al.*, 1977) examined the effect of 15 min of pharmacist drug counselling just before geriatric patients were discharged. We found a substantial improvement in both drug compliance and drug regimen comprehension. This improvement was seen even in confused patients. The effect of counselling was most marked after 1 week but declined only marginally over 12 weeks. So the evidence suggests that regimen education gives variable results. No study has assessed the benefits beyond 3 months. It may well be that instruction gives only short-term benefit, declining slowly as the months roll on.

One method of drug education is to give a drug reminder chart or leaflet. Ley *et al.* (1976a) showed a modest improvement in compliance with an easy-read leaflet on taking the drug. Gabriel *et al.* (1977) showed that a daily dose-reminder chart substantially improved compliance in a fairly elderly group of hypertensives. This well-designed study documented that the effect persisted for at least 2 months. So written reminders may well be useful, although we are unsure of the duration of their effect.

Package inserts have also been proposed to educate patients about their drug, with details of how to take the drug, how to store it, side-effects, etc. (Hermann *et al.*, 1978). No studies have been made of their effectiveness.

Getting the message across more effectively

Doctors can take advantage of studies by educational psychologists on how best to get patients to understand and remember facts given to them. These studies have been reviewed by Ley *et al.* (1976b), and the basic conclusions are summarized in Table 14.3. These conclusions merit a few further comments.

Give instructions and advice early in the interview. Facts given in the first third of the interview are more likely to be remembered (Ley, 1972).

Stress the importance of the advice you give. Patients have been shown to forget about half the advice they have been given within 5 min of the interview (Ley *et al.*, 1973). Stressing an important point increases the chance of it being in the remembered half.

Use short words and short sentences. Most medical communications are too complicated for a substantial proportion of patients. Compliance has been shown to improve if written instructions are made more understandable (Ley *et al.*, 1976a) and this also appears to be the case for oral instructions.

Table 14.3   Suggestions for improving doctor–patient communication

Give instructions and advice early in the interview
Stress the importance of the advice you give
Use short words and short sentences
Arrange your advice into clear categories
Repeat the important advice
Give specific and exact advice rather than general recommendations

Arrange advice in clear categories. This can increase recall by up to 50% (Ley *et al.*, 1973).

Repeat advice. This fundamental tenet of education can sometimes be forgotten in the heat of a consultation.

Give specific exact advice rather than general recommendations. The more specific the advice is, the more powerful the effect is on retention and behaviour (Ley, 1975).

These suggestions have been proven individually in experimental settings and have been tried collectively in practice. The suggestions were incorporated into a booklet given to dieters to help achieve weight loss. It substantially improved weight loss compared to a standard booklet (Ley, 1976). The suggestions were given to a group of somewhat sceptical general practitioners to use during consultations (Ley *et al.*, 1976b). After they used the suggestions their patients remembered 27% more of the statements they made. This improvement in communication was seen with every doctor and seemed independent of his initial competence in communication. The greatest improvement was seen in geriatric patients—they remembered 52% more. So applying these suggestions is particularly important in getting the message across to the elderly.

Educating the doctor

Like many other aspects of medical care, compliance faces the problem of 'how to motivate the motivators' (Rouillon, 1972). But would teaching doctors about compliance make any difference to their patients' compliance? In an important study Inui *et al.* (1976) gave tutorials to hospital medical staff on hypertension and stressed that the probability of non-compliance was very high if blood pressure control was poor. These tutorials improved the incidence of good compliance in their patients from 32% to 61%. Compliance was measured by surprise home pill counts, so should be reliable. Also, the proportion of well-controlled patients (diastolic ≤100 mm Hg) rose from 36% to 69%. This improvement in control lasted for at least 6 months. So educating doctors about compliance really does seem to work.

Modifying the regimen

Reducing the number of drugs

Virtually all reports agree that compliance falls off as the number of prescribed drugs increases. This appears to be especially true for old people. Many studies have noted that compliance falls particularly sharply if three or more drugs are prescribed. A finer point is whether a combination drug tablet gives better compliance than two or more individual tablets. This has been reviewed by Haynes *et al.* (1977), who found the evidence equivocal. So combination tablets do not automatically improve compliance. Nevertheless, the overall conclusion is clear: cut down the number of drugs and never give more than three if at all possible.

Reducing the frequency of dosing

Advertisers have recently taken to claiming that tablets taken once daily will give better compliance than those taken in more frequent doses. Unfortunately, the effect of dose frequency on compliance is not well documented. The few studies available are old, and their methods can be criticized. Gatley (1968) found a smooth steep decline from 67% compliance (once daily) to 22% compliance (four times daily). But patient numbers were small (only three patients in the once-daily group), duration of courses varied substantially, and the 20% of patients who failed to complete the study were excluded. Porter (1969) found that compliance among pregnant women taking iron was significantly better on once-daily therapy than on thrice-daily therapy. Even so, the thrice-daily group consumed four times as much iron as the once-daily group. Neither of these groups had random allocation, nor were they controlled for other factors such as level of supervision, length of drug course, number of other drugs, etc. Two other studies (Ayd, 1972; Clinite and Kabat, 1976) point to similar conclusions, but the methods also have problems. On the other hand, well-conducted trials by Hulka *et al.* (1975) and Parkin *et al.* (1976) have shown no effect of dose frequency on compliance. The effect of dose frequency on comprehension has been studied only by Hulka *et al.* (1975), who found that increased dose frequency brought increasing non-comprehension. Thus the evidence that less frequent dosing brings compliance benefits is far from convincing. We still need a really well-organized trial to test this idea.

Using alternative drugs

The evidence tends to suggest that changing to an alternative drug in a given disease produces little compliance benefit (Haynes *et al.*, 1977). This idea has, however, only been assessed in a few studies, so further work might clarify this point.

Using supervised parenteral administration

If a drug can be made in a parenteral formulation which is long-acting, it can be given directly by medical or paramedical staff. Any lapse whatsoever in compliance is immediately obvious—failing to turn up for an injection—and corrective action can be taken. In theory this method should be an excellent way of improving compliance. In practice it has proved to be consistently successful. Long-acting depot penicillins have been tried for both short-term treatment of acute streptococcal pharyngitis (Colcher and Bass, 1972) and long-term prophylaxis of rheumatic fever (Feinstein *et al.*, 1959, 1968). In all three studies the regimens were well tolerated by patients and produced substantial improvements in clinical outcome.

Twice-weekly supervised chemotherapy has long been used in the treatment of tuberculosis. The wide variety of suitable regimens has been summarized by Macdonald (1979). Fox (1968) has concluded that these regimens are as effective as the best daily regimens and has suggested that physicians should and will use these supervised regimens more frequently in the treatment of tuberculosis (Fox, 1971).

The greatest triumph of supervised parenteral medication has undoubtedly been in the use of long-acting phenothiazines in schizophrenia. In a rigorous study Johnson and Freeman (1972) found that changing to intramuscular fluphenazine from oral phenothiazines reduced the number of hospital admissions for relapse by 26% and the number of days spent in hospital by 52%.

All the trials above have used unselected groups of patients. But is this type of regimen effective on patients specifically selected for being non-compliant? Two studies have used twice-weekly parenteral regimens to treat unco-operative alcoholics for tuberculosis (Onstad *et al.*, 1970; Hudson and Sbarbaro, 1973). The cure rates were 98% and 99%—superb results in these highly awkward patients. So the method works well in even the most difficult clinical situations.

How do patients react to the inconvenience of attending for treatment? A study in Lancashire (Lal, 1969) showed that patients given the choice preferred twice-weekly supervised treatment for tuberculosis to daily self-treatment. A very large Czech study (Polansky, 1970) also showed this to be the case. The patient's ability to choose his type of therapy may well create an informal contract between the doctor and patient which improves compliance—'I did actually ask for this sort of treatment, so I suppose I had better stick to it.'

Would supervised intermittent oral therapy work? Sbarbaro and Hudson (1974) commented on a marked improvement in 'patient acceptance' of the medication after switching from parenteral to oral twice-weekly supervised antituberculous chemotherapy in non-compliant patients. However, 'patient acceptance' was not defined. The missed appointment rate rose from 4.5% (parenteral) to 6.9% (oral) and patients often asked why they could not take the pills home with them. This appears to be the only study assessing compliance with long-term supervised intermittent oral regimens. It suggests that this method could be successful if suitable drugs were available. Further evidence that supervised administration rather than the parenteral route is the key to success comes from the appalling compliance rates for self-injected insulin (Watkins *et al.*, 1967). It looks as if supervised administration of long-acting drugs (oral or parenteral) markedly improves compliance. The problem is that so few drugs are presently available in long-acting formulations. Fitzgerald (1976) has pointed out that the root of this is manufacturers' fears of commercial failure caused by side-effects rather than insuperable problems in developing long-acting forms. Side-effects have not been a particular problem in long-acting phenothiazines for schizophrenia or other such drugs. The market for a once-monthly injected drug, for example, for hypertension would be gigantic. Development of long-acting drugs could be a great boon to the patient and also to the drug firms.

Increasing medical supervision

More frequent contact between doctor and patient might itself improve compliance. Several studies have looked at this. In most of them it is difficult to isolate increased supervision from other factors, but they mainly show a sizeable improvement in compliance. Broadly speaking, the more often the patients are seen the better they comply.

Always seeing the same doctor

Surprisingly, most studies have not shown any improvement in compliance on always seeing the same doctor, rather than a stream of different doctors.

Table 14.4   Methods for improving compliance

Effective	Probably effective	Not effective
Patient education about regimen*	Patient education about regimen	Patient education about disease
Reducing number of drugs	Written instructions	Using alternative drugs
Using supervised parenteral medication	Reducing dose frequency	Always seeing the same doctor
Measuring drug levels		Using special containers
Educating the doctor about compliance		

* Short-term regimens only

Measuring blood levels of drugs

Facilities for measuring blood levels are widely available for a range of oral drugs including digoxin, anti-epileptics, theophyllines, tricyclic anti-depressants, and lithium. At least five studies have shown that measuring blood levels produces an improvement in compliance (as well as in therapeutic efficiency). Outcome was also improved in the two studies where it was assessed separately. The problems of sample timing, therapeutic ranges, etc. have been discussed in Chapter 11. Measuring blood levels is one of the most effective ways of proving that the patient is getting and taking the right dose.

Dispensing in special containers

No study has yet shown any improvement in long-term compliance from dispensing drugs in special containers or in packs aimed at assisting compliance. Our own study (Macdonald *et al.*, 1977) showed that a pill-wheel dispenser actually reduced compliance.

CONCLUSIONS

Of the many ways of improving compliance only a few are worth their salt. These are summarized in Table 14.4. For short-term regimens, giving exact detailed spoken and written instructions on how to take the regimen is best; very simple and very effective.

Other more complicated but effective ways are to give supervised parenteral treatment, use individual patient calendars, and follow-up supervision by paramedical staff.

For long-term regimens, getting good compliance is distinctly more difficult. Cutting down the number of drugs prescribed, measuring blood levels, and giving supervised therapy where possible are the most effective methods. Clear instructions at interview, frequent patient visits, and educating the doctor about compliance all have a role to play.

REFERENCES

Ayd, F. J. Jr (1972) Once-a-day neuroleptic and tricyclic antidepressant therapy. *Int. Drug Ther. Newsletter*, **7**, 33–40.
Beanland, W. A. (1975) A new approach to labelling. *Pharmacist J.*, **214**, 507.
Bowen, R. G. *et al.* (1961) Effects of organised instruction for patients with the diagnosis of diabetes mellitus. *Nurs. Res.*, **10**, 151–9.
Clinite, J. and Kabat, H. (1976) Improving patient compliance. *J. Am. Pharm. Assoc.*, **16**, 74–6 and 85.

238

Colcher, I. S. and Bass, J. W. (1972) Penicillin treatment of streptococcal pharyngitis: a comparison of schedules and the role of specific counselling. *JAMA*, **222**, 657–9.

Cole, P. and Emmanuel (1971) Drug consultation: its significance to the discharged hospital patient and its relevance as a role for the pharmacist. *Am. J. Hosp. Pharm.*, **28**, 954–60.

Etzwiler, D. D. and Robb, J. R. (1972) Evaluation of programmed education among juvenile diabetics and their families. *Diabetes*, **21**, 967–71.

Feinstein, A. R. *et al.* (1959) A controlled study of three methods of prophylaxis against streptococcal infection in a population of rheumatic children. (II) Results of the first three years of the study, including methods for evaluating the maintenance of oral prophylaxis. *New Engl. J. Med.*, **260**, 697–702.

Feinstein, A. R. *et al.* (1968) Prophylaxis of recurrent rheumatic fever. *JAMA*, **206**, 565–8.

Fitzgerald, J. D. (1976) The influence of the medication on compliance with therapeutic regimens. In D. L. Sackett and R. B. Haynes (eds), *Compliance with Therapeutic Regimens*, pp. 119–28. Johns Hopkins University Press, Baltimore.

Fox, W. (1968) The John Barnwell Lecture: changing concepts in the chemotherapy of pulmonary tuberculosis. *Am. Rev. Resp. Dis.*, **97**, 767–90.

Fox, W. (1971) General considerations in intermittent drug therapy of pulmonary tuberculosis. *Postgrad. Med. J.*, **47**, 729–36.

Gabriel, M. *et al.* (1977) Improved patient compliance through use of a daily drug reminder chart. *Am. J. Publ. Health*, **67**, 968–9.

Gatley, M. S. (1968) To be taken as directed. *J. Roy. Coll. Gen. Pract.*, **16**, 39–44.

Haynes, R. *et al.* (1977) Manipulation of the therapeutic regimen to improve patient compliance: conceptions and misconceptions. *Clin. Pharmacol. Ther.*, **22**, 125–30.

Hecht, A. B. (1974) Improving medication compliance by teaching outpatients. *Nurs. Forum*, **13**, 112–29.

Hermann, F. *et al.* (1978) Package inserts for prescribed medicines: what minimum information do patients need? *Brit. Med. J.*, **2**, 1132–5.

Hudson, L. D. and Sbarbaro, J. A. (1973) Twice-weekly tuberculosis chemotherapy. *JAMA*, **223**, 139.

Hulka, B. *et al.* (1975) Medication use and misuse: physician–patient discrepancies. *J. Chron. Dis.*, **28**, 7–21.

Inui, T. *et al.* (1976) Improved outcomes in hypertension after physician tutorials. *Ann. Intern. Med.*, **84**, 646–51.

Johnson, D. and Freeman, H. (1972) Long-acting tranquilisers. *Practitioner*, **208**, 395–400.

Lal, S. (1969) Patients' preference of drugs in the treatment of tuberculosis. *Tubercle*, **50**, 269.

Ley, P. (1972) Primacy, rated importance, and the recall of medical statements. *J. Health Soc. Behav.*, **13**, 311–17.

Ley, P. (1975) The use of techniques and findings from social and experimental psychology to improve doctor–patient communications. In *Health Education and Primary Care: Conference Report*, pp. 14–35. Department of Community Medicine and Leeds Polytechnic, Leeds.

Ley, P. (1976) Towards better doctor–patient communications. In Bennett, A. E. (ed), *Communications in Medicine*, pp. 75–98. Oxford University Press, London.

Ley, P. *et al.* (1973) A method for increasing patients' recall of information presented by doctors. *Psychol. Med.*, **3**, 217–20.

Ley, P. *et al.* (1976a) A method for decreasing patients' medication errors. *Psychol. Med.*, **6**, 599–601.

Ley, P. *et al.* (1976b) Improving doctor–patient communication in general practice. *J. roy. Coll. Gen. Pract.*, **26**, 720–4.

Linkewich, J. A. *et al.* (1974) The effect of packaging and instruction on outpatient compliance with medication regimens. *Drug Intell. Clin. Pharm.*, **8**, 10–15.

Macdonald, E. T. *et al.* (1977) Improving drug compliance after hospital discharge. *Brit. Med. J.*, **2**, 618–21.

Macdonald, J. B. (1979) The origin of treatment failure in tuberculosis: a clinical study of the development of drug resistance. M.D. Thesis, University of Cambridge, pp. 162–8.

Malahy, B. (1966) The effect of instruction and labelling on the number of medication errors made by patients at home. *Am. J. Hosp. Pharm.*, **23**, 283–92.

Onstad, G. D. *et al.* (1970) Posthospital chemotherapy of the unreliable patient. *Am. Rev. Resp. Dis.*, **101**, 258–64.

Parkin, D. M. *et al.* (1976) Deviation from prescribed drug treatment after discharge from hospital. *Brit. Med. J.*, **2**, 686–8.

Polansky, F. (1970) Trial of sanatorium treatment including a comparison of standard and intermittent continuation chemotherapy. *Bull. Int. Union. Tuberc.*, **43**, 295.

Porter, A. M. (1969) Drug defaulting in a general practice. *Brit. Med. J.*, **1**, 218–22.

Rehder, T. *et al.* (1980) Improving compliance by counselling and pill container. *Am. J. Hosp. Pharm.*, **37**, 379–85.

Rouillon, A. (1972) What is motivation? *Bull. Int. Union Tuberc.*, **47**, 69–72.

Sackett, D. L. *et al.* (1975) Randomised clinical trial of strategies for improving medication compliance in primary hypertension. *Lancet*, **1**, 1205–7.

Sbarbaro, J. A. and Hudson, L. D. (1974) High dose ethambutol: an oral alternate to intermittent chemotherapy. *Am. Rev. Resp. Dis.*, **10**, 91–4.

Sharpe, T. R. and Mikeal, R. L. (1974) Patient compliance with antibiotic regimens. *Am. J. Hosp. Pharm.*, **31**, 479–84.

Tagliacozzo, D. M. *et al.* (1974) Nurse intervention and patient behaviour. *Am. J. Publ. Health*, **64**, 596–603.

Watkins, J. D. *et al.* (1967) A study of diabetic patients at home. *Am. J. Publ. Health*, **57**, 452–9.

Index